THE
7 STAGES
OF
HEALING

A Guide to Recovery After
Surgery, Illness, or Trauma

Kenna Kaylee

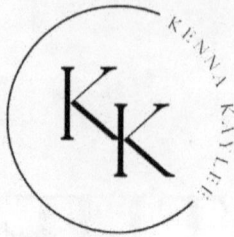

ISBN: 979-8-9933043-0-4

First Edition

Where scars mark the body's healing, emotions remain unseen, carving their stories within, and waiting for courage to uncover them. We learn quickly how to hide what hurts, but real recovery begins the moment we stop pretending and allow ourselves to feel what we've buried.

Contents

AUTHOR'S NOTE

Nine years ago, I began writing words I never imagined would be shared. At the time, I had no vision, no clear direction, only pages filled with raw reflections as I watched my ex-husband face a devastating accident and loss that shattered our lives. Those pages were never meant to become anything more than a place to release the pain I carried.

What followed was a dark season of divorce and desperate attempts to numb myself. I convinced myself that escape was the only way out. But the more I tried to silence the hurt, the more I lost sight of the very person I had once been. Instead of healing, I was burying my grief so deeply that it touched every part of my life. What I thought was survival was really surrender, and it left me emptier than before.

It was not until I began the painful work of facing my grief, my failures, and my brokenness that I slowly found the strength to begin again. Healing did not come quickly or neatly. It came in waves, with setbacks and small victories that, at the time, felt impossible to hold onto. But as I poured my hurt and observations onto paper, I began to see patterns. The stages we walk through when life as we know it collapses: pain, fear, anger, sadness, guilt, acceptance, and finally empowerment.

Even now, years later, my ex remains in my life. Despite everything, I will always be the first to care for him. That is part of my story too, that compassion can survive even the deepest breaks, and that healing often asks us to hold more than one truth at once.

As a nurse, I have cared for countless patients and families walking through these same struggles. I have watched people battle their way back from surgeries, illnesses, and traumas that seemed insurmountable. I have seen caregivers wear exhaustion on their faces yet show up every day with unshakable love. And years later, I found myself reliving the journey again as my fiancé nearly lost his life, forcing me to face the stages all over once more.

This book is not a manual or a roadmap. It is a reflection of the truth I have lived and witnessed: healing is not linear. It is messy, painful, unpredictable, and deeply personal. But within it lies a strength you may not yet know you have. No matter what you are going through, whether surgery, illness, or trauma, your story matters. You are not broken. You are not alone. And there is light at the end of this tunnel.

For the patients fighting for their lives, for the survivors who carry their scars, for the caregivers who hold them up when they cannot stand, and for anyone walking through the vulnerable recovery of elective surgery, this book is for you. Healing, no matter its cause, is never a straight path. Setbacks are not failures; they are part of the process. My hope is that these words remind you that the stages are all normal, and that moving through them does not make you weak, it makes you human. May you find comfort, validation, and strength in knowing you are not alone, and may you discover that empowerment is not the end of healing but the beginning of a new life.

With compassion,

Kenna 🖤

INTRODUCTION

The beeping of the monitor was steady, but my heart was not.

I gripped his hand, waiting for movement, a flicker, anything to show me he was still in there. His eyelids fluttered open, groggy from the anesthesia, his eyes darting around the sterile hospital room. And then, it happened, his breathing hitched, his fingers clenched mine in desperation, and his voice, hoarse and shaky, whispered the words that would change everything.

"I can't move my legs.

The air left my lungs.

A thousand thoughts flooded my mind. Maybe he was still numb from the surgery. Maybe it was the medication. Or maybe no, it wasn't. I saw it in his eyes, the way panic clawed at his throat like a scream he couldn't release. I had seen this before, caring for patients just like him, but nothing, and I mean *nothing*, prepares you for the moment when the person lying in that bed is someone you love.

I swallowed the fear rising in my chest and did what I had done so many times before. I softened my voice, steadied my hands, and became the nurse in the room. "It's okay," I said, the words feeling empty even as I spoke them. "You're safe. We'll figure this out." But even as I reassured him, my own heart pounded with uncertainty.

Just a few doors down, a fiancé lay motionless, blinking up at the ceiling, his mind racing as the doctor's words echoed in his head.

"You almost died."

His appendix had ruptured, and the infection was spreading fast, tipping him into sepsis. He had no idea how close he had come to not waking up. Now, the real battle began. His road to recovery would be long. Weeks filled with exhaustion, months spent rebuilding strength, and years of wondering if his body would ever feel the same again.

Somewhere else in this same hospital, a mother rested in bed, staring out the window, afraid to move after her C-section. Down the hall, a teenager fresh out of ACL surgery felt the first wave of post-op nausea crash over him.

A few miles away, a woman who had previously lost 200 pounds woke up from skin removal surgery, her body aching, her mind racing with the weight of what had just happened. After years of feeling trapped in skin that no longer felt like her own, she had finally shed it. But the reality of recovery was setting in.

Across town, a young woman opened her eyes, her back aching unlike anything she'd felt before. She had lived with chronic back pain for years because her large breasts were weighing her down physically (and emotionally). Now, after her long-awaited breast reduction, she wondered how long it would take before she could feel like herself again.

Across the country, a woman sat at home, afraid to look in the mirror, her face swollen and bruised from a cosmetic procedure she had waited years to afford.

These are different stories and diverse bodies, yet they share a raw vulnerability. Whether you're healing from life-saving surgery or an elective procedure you've opted for, whether your healing process started with an accident or a diagnosis, the emotional phases are the same. Your body may be healing for various reasons, but your mind and heart take the same journey through pain, fear, doubt, anger, sadness, and then to acceptance, and ultimately, empowerment.

Pain is a subjective experience and cannot be measured by comparisons. A spinal cord injury doesn't diminish the pain felt by a woman recovering from a facelift, just as a broken toe doesn't lessen the seriousness of a broken femur. Waking up from an infection that nearly killed you doesn't make the agony of waking up from any surgery, elective or not, any less overwhelming.

Suffering is suffering. Healing is healing. No matter the circumstance, the recovery process has the power to shake your identity, test your patience, and challenge you in ways you never expected.

That's why this journey matters, and why this book exists.

But this is what no one tells you about healing. Your body might recover, but your heart and mind have minds of their own. While surgeons watch for surgical wounds and vital signs, there's an entire emotional process unfolding beneath the surface, one that takes place in seven predictable steps that almost everyone experiences but almost no one talks about.

This book will take you through those seven steps of healing that nobody tells you about, because healing your body is only half the battle. Regardless of whether you're healing from life-saving surgery, a terrible accident, an elective surgery you decided on, cancer treatment, a broken limb, or living with a chronic illness, the emotional steps are the same. Your body may be recovering from various reasons, yet your mind and heart take the same journey.

If you're in a hospital bed as you read this, if you're confined to your couch at home, or if you're cradling someone you love through healing, this book is for you. You'll know why that crushing wave of sadness washes over you when you least expect it, why anger burns so fiercely even when you choose to have your procedure, and why healing often takes a step backward instead of forward.

Most of all, you'll know that every confusing, overwhelming emotion you're experiencing isn't a sign that something's wrong. It's proof that healing is happening, even when it doesn't feel like it.

1

<u>Pain</u>

Shock & Discomfort

The first thing she felt was fire.

Not the dull ache she had braced herself for. Not the tightness the doctor had mentioned. This was pure fire deep, unrelenting, wrapping around her body like a vise and spreading hot coals beneath her skin.

She tried to move, a decision she regretted. The pain clawed through her ribs, sharp and consuming, stealing the air from her lungs.

Her mind raced. *What the hell did I do to myself?*

She instinctively reached up, but her arms felt like dead weight. Her fingertips grazed against something stiff and unfamiliar. Bandages, thick and unyielding, were suffocating her body.

Panic set in.

She gasped, but the simple act of inhaling sent another bolt of agony through her ribs. The room blurred. Her body wasn't hers anymore. It was something else, something broken. Something she had *chosen.*

"Breathe," she urged herself, but each breath came in shallow, ragged gasps.

She had waited years for this. Saved up for it. Dreamed of how she would feel afterward. But this? This wasn't part of the plan.

She could still hear herself laughing in the mirror the night before, twisting side to side, imagining how different she'd look.

"This is it," she had said to her best friend, grinning as she took one last "before" picture.

She had scrolled through Instagram, where she had found those perfect post-op glow-ups of women smiling in their sleek compression garments, raving about how it was the best decision they had ever made.

She had imagined herself weeks from now, standing taller and more confident. Her surgeon had reassured her that it was going to be a smooth recovery.

"A little tightness, some soreness, but nothing you can't handle," he had said.

That morning, she had practically skipped into the clinic, excited and nervous, but ready. Now, hours later, reality hit her like a train.

A soft voice cut through the haze. A nurse hovered nearby, checking the monitors. "How's your pain?"

"I don't know," she whispered, her throat dry, her words barely audible. The truth was, she struggled to describe what she was feeling.

Pain wasn't supposed to feel this overwhelming. It surrounded her, inescapable and unrelenting. The pressure in her chest. The sharpness in her ribs. The constant, nauseating ache radiating from her skin.

"It'll get better soon," the nurse reassured her, adjusting her IV. *Would it?*

She had read the pamphlets. Watched the videos. No one had warned her about *this,* the way pain could swallow you whole and make you second-guess everything.

As she shifted, a fresh wave of agony ripped through her. Her stomach churned, and tears burned behind her eyes.

A creeping thought slithered into her mind.

Did I make a mistake?

WHAT IS PAIN?

Pain is the body's alarm system, signaling that something has changed and needs attention. Whether from surgery, injury, or illness, pain is a biological response designed to protect and heal you. In the first hours and days after a medical event, pain can be intense, deep, or even suffocating. But understanding why it happens can help transform fear into reassurance.

From the moment a procedure ends, the body goes into high alert. Surgery, no matter how controlled, is still considered "trauma" in the eyes of the nervous system. Nerve endings, blood vessels, and tissues have been disrupted, triggering an immediate chain reaction of responses.

The brain receives distress signals from the affected area, translating them into pain. In response, the immune system floods the site with healing cells, causing redness, swelling, and heat. Fluids build up around tissues, exerting pressure on nerves and creating a throbbing and tight feeling as the body adjusts. Muscles instinctively tense up to protect the wounded area, increasing discomfort.

All of these reactions are completely normal.

Pain after surgery is not a sign that something is wrong. It's a sign that the body is actively working to repair itself.

Many people underestimate post-surgical pain because surgery is a planned procedure rather than an unexpected injury. But the experience of pain after an operation can differ significantly from initial expectations.

Acute injury can result from an unexpected fall, accident, or impact, often accompanied by a sudden, sharp sensation, followed by shock or adrenaline. Post-surgical pain is usually deeper, more widespread, and lasts longer. It's often accompanied by swelling, stiffness, and a delayed reaction as anesthesia wears off.

Even if you're mentally prepared for pain, your body will still react to surgery as if it were trauma. It's okay if it feels more intense than you expected.

Pain isn't limited to the surgical site and is affected by three major factors: inflammation, swelling, and nerve sensitivity.

Inflammation is the body's natural response to injury and healing. White blood cells are sent to the affected area, causing redness, warmth, and swelling that intensifies pain.

Swelling increases pressure on surrounding tissues, nerves, and blood vessels, making even the lightest touch unbearable.

Nerve sensitivity varies depending on the procedure and individual pain thresholds. Surgery can irritate or temporarily damage nerves, resulting in tingling, burning, or numbness in specific areas.

This is why pain can feel unpredictable. One moment, it's dull and throbbing, and the next, a sudden movement can send a sharp, stabbing sensation. The nervous system is recalibrating to make sense of what happened.

Pain is more than just a physical sensation. It's an emotional experience. The brain doesn't separate physical pain from emotional distress the way we think it does.

Harvard Medical School research indicates that chronic pain and emotional distress use the same neural pathways in the brain, the anterior cingulate cortex, and the insula. Dr. Naomi Eisenberger's seminal work at UCLA proved that social rejection uses the same brain areas as physical pain, which is why emotional hurt actually "hurts" (UCLA Department of Psychology, n.d.). Furthermore, research published in the Journal of Pain Research found that patients who are aware of the neurological connection between physical and emotional pain experience 23% improved pain management outcomes and reduced anxiety during recovery (Lumley et al., 2012).

The same regions of the brain that process physical pain also process heartbreak, grief, and trauma. Emotional stress can worsen pain by increasing muscle tension and inflammation. Fear, anxiety, and sadness can intensify physical symptoms, making pain feel more severe and harder to manage.

This is why post-operative pain can feel overwhelming both in the body and mind. It's okay if pain makes you feel emotional. If you find yourself crying, feeling frustrated, or even regretting your decision, you're not weak. You're human.

Pain means healing, not failure. Your experience is valid, regardless of the size of the procedure. Emotional and physical pain are connected, and healing requires patience and self-compassion.

Dr. Joseph LeDoux, a neuroscientist who has studied fear conditioning, explains that the amygdala (our brain's alarm system) doesn't differentiate between perceived and real danger (LeDoux, 2024). In recovery, this primitive survival mechanism interprets every new sensation as a possible threat. Brain imaging research demonstrates that anticipatory anxiety can actually heighten pain perception, setting up a self-reinforcing cycle (Robb-Dover, 2023). But Stanford's Pain Management Center research discovered that patients who regularly practice grounding techniques and mindfulness demonstrate reduced amygdala activation in as little as two weeks (Martin, 2024).

Understanding your body's healing process reduces fear. This stage is temporary. Time unlocks your body's natural tendency to repair, restore, and recover.

Though this stage can seem never-ending, pain doesn't last forever. The next section will focus on how to manage pain effectively, including medications, natural relief methods, and mindset shifts.

WHY THIS STAGE HAPPENS

Pain serves as the brutal gatekeeper to recovery, the body's way of demanding that we pay attention.. The moment trauma occurs, the nervous system fires off distress signals to alert the brain that something is wrong. The body doesn't process these signals rationally. Instead, it prioritizes survival above all else.

Immediately after trauma, inflammation kicks in, a necessary but excruciating part of healing. The immune system floods the injured area with white blood cells, fluids, and proteins to repair damaged tissues. This response causes swelling, stiffness, and an intense throbbing sensation that makes every movement feel like punishment. Pain is like a battle inside your body as it fights to protect and rebuild itself.

Pain is worst in the beginning due to the heightened sensitivity of the nervous system. After surgery or injury, pain receptors are on high alert, amplifying every ache, sting, and burn. The body is trying to prevent further damage by limiting movement, signaling the need for rest and recovery. Unfortunately, this heightened sensitivity makes everything feel unbearable, even when you're doing exactly what you're supposed to be doing.

On top of that, the body is also in a state of shock. If anesthesia was used, a chemical and neurological rebound effect takes place as the system wakes up. The transition from numbness to feeling everything at once is jarring. Pain feels more shocking than expected, not only because of the injury itself but because the body is recalibrating after being in an altered state.

The brain interprets pain, labeling it as a threat and initiating a fight-or-flight response, flooding the system with adrenaline and cortisol. The heart races and breathing becomes shallow as panic sets in. The more fear that is felt, the more tense the body becomes, increasing the perception of suffering. Anxiety makes pain feel sharper, more consuming, and more unbearable, creating a loop of physical and emotional distress that feeds off each other.

The hardest part of this stage is that it feels like it will never end. Pain distorts the perception of time, making minutes feel like hours, hours like days. The mind spirals into a cycle of doubt, second-guessing everything. This isn't a sign of weakness. This is biology at work.

Pain will try to convince you that you'll never feel normal again, but this is a lie.

Pain is a transition, not a permanent state. The worst of it happens when the body is doing the most intense repair work. As inflammation subsides and nerve sensitivity decreases, pain begins to change as the body adjusts. It might shift, dull, or come in waves, but it won't remain at this unbearable peak forever.

Reframing pain is essential. Instead of seeing it as endless suffering, see it as evidence that the body is doing exactly what it's supposed to do. You do not have to be fearless. You just have to keep moving forward, one moment at a time.

COMMON STRUGGLES IN THIS STAGE

Pain affects every aspect of life, from daily routines to emotional stability. In the early stages of healing, many people struggle with more than the discomfort itself. It's not just about enduring it but also learning to navigate the limitations that come with it. And let's be honest, some of those limitations are straight-up ridiculous.

One of the most common struggles is how much worse the pain feels compared to expectations. No matter how much preparation goes into a procedure, nothing fully prepares the body or mind for the reality of the healing process. The deep, aching, sometimes stabbing pain can be overwhelming, especially in the first few days when it feels like there will be no relief in sight. The expectation of "manageable discomfort" quickly turns into "Holy shit. Am I dying?" and suddenly, that post-op care packet seems like a pack of lies.

Dependence on others can be just as difficult to accept as the pain itself. Things that once felt automatic, such as getting out of bed, showering, or making a cup of coffee, now feel like Olympic-level challenges.. There's nothing like having to ask someone to pull up your pants or fetch you a snack because you're stuck in bed, feeling useless. Needing assistance with basic needs can leave you feeling helpless and vulnerable, especially if you're used to being independent. But right now, you are a baby bird in recovery. Let people take care of you.

Then comes the mirror moment. The first time you catch a

glimpse of yourself post-op. You're bruised, swollen, pale, and sporting the stylish hospital-chic look of tangled hair, dry lips, and the faint scent of medical tape. Nobody warns you that recovery comes with looking like you got hit by a truck. Even if the surgery was elective, there's a good chance that instead of feeling fabulous, you feel like a bloated corpse dragged through a battlefield. It's temporary, but at the moment, it's hard to believe.

Sleep, or rather the complete lack of it, becomes a struggle instead of a source of rest. Finding a comfortable position feels impossible when every small movement sends waves of pain through the body. Shifting slightly can bring a sharp jolt of agony, making it hard to relax. Just as exhaustion takes over, you're rudely awakened again by pain, stiffness, or medication side effects. And if that doesn't do it, the hospital or home recovery noises will., Imagine the hum of medical equipment, a TV droning in the background, or a well-meaning loved one snoring next to you while you plot their demise.

Movement restrictions add another layer of frustration. The natural instinct is to return to normal as soon as possible, but the body is not ready. Simple actions, such as standing up, rolling over, or even taking a deep breath, can feel monumental. Every tiny motion requires far too much effort. Walking to the bathroom feels like an expedition to Mount Everest, minus the inspiring views.

And speaking of the bathroom, let's talk about constipation. If there's one thing that should be in bold, capital letters on every post-op instruction sheet, it should be, *"You will not poop for days!"* No one prepares you for the fact that between anesthesia, pain medication, and lounging around, your digestive system essentially goes on strike. You'll be there for twenty minutes, clutching the sink, having entire conversations with your own intestines.

"Please. I'm begging you! I've done prune juice, I've walked laps around the house, I've taken yoga poses that probably broke my surgical restrictions!"

When it does finally happen, you'll text your partner as if you've won the lottery.

At first, it's just discomfort. Then it becomes a mission. It's an experience no one prepares you for, but every recovering patient knows it all too well.

Medications add their own set of struggles. While they help manage pain, they can also leave you feeling groggy, nauseated, or straight-up loopy. One minute, you're nodding off mid-sentence, and the next, you're deep in thought about the meaning of life while staring at the wall. Conversations become a challenge when your brain is ten seconds behind real-time events. The balance between pain relief and feeling like yourself again is delicate, and in those early days, it's completely normal to feel like an extra in a zombie movie.

All of these struggles are normal. They don't mean that something is wrong or that healing is not happening. This phase of recovery requires patience, allowing the body the time it needs to heal. Frustration, exhaustion, and even moments of doubt are part of the process. The key is to remember that these struggles are temporary. Your body is working hard, even when it feels like no progress is being made. Healing is happening, even during the hardest moments. And yes, eventually, you will poop again.

RECOVERY STRATEGIES IN THIS STAGE

Pain is dramatic. It doesn't gently tap you on the shoulder and ask for attention. No, it kicks the door in, flips over the furniture, and demands to be the center of your world. But just because pain is loud doesn't mean it gets to be in charge. There are ways to get ahead of it, manage it, and remind it that you're the one calling the shots.

Managing pain is more than just about taking medication and waiting for relief to kick in. It's about using every tool available to make sure pain doesn't own you. You can take control, get ahead of the pain instead of reacting to it, and work toward a recovery that's not just one long, miserable endurance test.

Pain meds are not the enemy. Let's just start there. For some reason, people get weird about taking medication after surgery, as if they need to prove how tough they are by suffering through it. There's no trophy for pain tolerance, and no one is handing out awards for gritting your teeth and refusing relief. If your doctor prescribed pain medication, take it as directed and don't feel guilty about it.

Pain meds work by blocking signals to the brain, helping to turn down the volume on the chaos happening in your body. They won't erase pain completely, but they can take the edge off enough so you can rest, move, and not feel like you're starring in your own personal horror movie.

What pain meds cannot do is fix everything. They are one tool in a much bigger pain management strategy. The goal is to manage the pain, not erase it completely, because pain is part of healing. You cannot be totally numb and expect to heal properly. The key is staying ahead, not letting pain get so bad that you're practically bargaining with the universe for relief.

Now, let's talk about the fear of addiction because it's real. Pain meds are not meant to be a long-term solution. If you're taking them as prescribed for post-op pain and tapering off when your body is ready, you won't suddenly wake up and find yourself starring in an after-school special about drug dependency. The key is listening to your body and knowing when the pain has diminished enough for you to switch to other pain relief methods.

Research in pain medicine shows that getting ahead of pain, rather than chasing it, is most effective One study found that patients who maintained consistent control over pain, rather than waiting for pain to be severe before taking medicine, required less medication overall and had better quality of sleep during recovery (Gauntlett-Gilbert, 2018).

If you're trying to cut back on pain meds or want to use every option available, there are non-medication strategies that can help take the sting out of recovery and make pain a little less of a diva. Here are some tips and tricks that may help:

- **Ice, heat, and elevation:** Ice is your best friend in the first few days after surgery. It reduces swelling, numbs pain, and makes everything feel a little less horrible. Later on, heat comes in handy, especially for easing stiff muscles. Elevation helps keep swelling down and prevents you from feeling like a human water balloon.
  - Applying ice wrapped in a thin towel for 15-20 minutes at a time can help numb acute pain and minimize swelling for the first 48-72 hours.
  - Don't apply ice directly to skin. You're healing, not attempting to get frostbite.
  - Once the initial inflammation subsides, heat is your friend. A heating pad set on low, a warm bath, or even that rice sock you nuked in the microwave can relax tight, sore muscles.

- Elevation is raising the swollen part above your heart whenever possible. Prop your leg up on pillows when you're watching TV, or sleep with an extra pillow if your upper body is what needs elevation.
- **Positioning for comfort:** If you're stuck in bed, find your sweet spot. You'll need the right pillows, proper propping of certain areas, and careful angle adjustments. All of these things make a difference. If you're uncomfortable, move things around until your body says, "Yes, this. This is the least terrible position possible."
- **Breathing techniques:** Sounds ridiculous, right? Like, how is breathing supposed to help when everything hurts? But it works. When you're in pain, your breathing gets shallow, and that makes everything worse. Deep, slow breaths tell your brain, "Hey, we are not dying. Calm down." This helps muscles relax, lowers your heart rate, and reduces the intensity of any aches.
- **Guided visualization:** Focus on anything else but your pain. Picture yourself somewhere calming. Imagine warmth, relief, and relaxation flooding your body. It might sound like nonsense, but your brain is powerful. When you focus on comfort instead of suffering, your body follows.

Keep in mind that while rest is important, too much rest will screw you over. It's a fine line. Your body needs downtime to heal, but lying in bed for days will make everything worse. Movement keeps blood flowing, prevents stiffness, and stops you from feeling like a bag of cement. It also prevents complications like blood clots, which are kind of a big deal. The goal is gentle, controlled movement, not running a marathon.

Start with the basics: shifting positions, wiggling your toes, bending and straightening your joints. It doesn't seem like much, but even subtle movements help your body recover faster. If your doctor has given you specific post-op exercises, do them, even if they suck. Your future self will thank you.

Pain wants you to think it's in charge. It wants you to feel helpless, stuck, and desperate. However, the truth is that you have options and control. Medication, non-medication techniques, movement, and mindset all work together to keep pain in check instead of letting it run the show.

Pain is loud, but you're stronger. This part of healing might be brutal, but it's also temporary. Keep throwing everything you have at it, and before you know it, you will be on the other side.

FINAL THOUGHTS

Healing pain comes and goes, gets better with medication, and gradually improves over time. Complication pain is relentless, sharp, worsening, or comes with other symptoms like swelling, fever, or nausea.

Think of healing pain like a bad roommate. Annoying, loud, always there, but predictable. Complication pain is like a house fire. Sudden, severe, and demanding immediate attention.

If something feels off, trust your gut. Doctors and nurses would rather tell you everything is okay than have you sit at home waiting while something gets worse.

Too many people suffer in silence after surgery because they are afraid of looking weak or being a burden. Let's clear this up right now: asking for more pain relief does not make you weak. It makes you responsible for your own recovery. If your pain is not being managed, you have every right to ask your doctor for more options.

There are multiple ways to manage pain beyond just one prescription. If your medication isn't effective, ask about alternatives. Different dosing, nerve blocks, pain patches, or even a combination of meds that might work better for your situation.

That said, pain management *does not* mean pain elimination. It's not safe, nor realistic, to be completely numb throughout recovery. Pain is a natural part of the healing process, and trying to eliminate it entirely can lead to more problems than it solves. The goal is to make it tolerable enough for you to rest, move, and heal. The goal *isn't* to check out from reality.

If you find yourself wanting to take extra medication to escape feeling anything at all, that's a sign to have a conversation with your doctor. There is a balance, and your medical team can help you find it.

Pain will try to convince you that it's permanent, unbearable, and in control. It will make you question everything. But here's the truth: pain is temporary, and you're in charge.

Know what is normal. Know when to call for help. Speak up if something is not working. And most importantly, remember that every day, every hour, every second that passes, your body is healing. It will not always feel like this. You are stronger than pain, and you decide how your story ends.

Pain is a storm. It will shake, break, and make you believe it will never end. But storms always pass.

JOURNAL PROMPT: Reframing Pain and Embracing Healing

Pain is a sign that your body is working hard to heal. Every ache and moment of discomfort is proof that you're moving forward, even when it doesn't feel like it. Shifting your mindset can help you find strength in the struggle.

1. How can I reframe my pain to focus on healing rather than suffering?
2. What part of the pain feels hardest to handle? Is it physical discomfort, exhaustion, or frustration with limitations?
3. How can I remind myself that pain is temporary and part of the healing process?
4. What thoughts or practices help me keep going when pain feels like too much?

Write it down. Take your time. Be honest. Let yourself acknowledge the challenge but also recognize the progress. Healing is happening, even in the hardest moments.

Instead of "This pain is unbearable," try "This pain is temporary, and each day brings relief." Instead of "I hate how weak I feel," remind yourself, "Rest is rebuilding, not weakness." Instead of "I will never feel normal again," focus on "Healing is happening, even when I can't see it.

2

Fear

Uncertainty & Anxiety

It had been a few days since surgery, and while the pain had settled into a dull, persistent ache, it felt more like a constant hum you can't shut off. He should have been feeling better by now. He should have been grateful that his body no longer felt like it had been run over by a semi. Instead of relief, something worse had moved in.

At first, it was just a stray thought. *Should it still hurt like this?* Then came the doubt. *Is this normal?* Then the paranoia. *What if it's not? What if something is really wrong?*

Now, he was lying in bed, stiff as a board, convinced that if he moved, something inside him might snap in half. Or explode. Or spectacularly fail in a way modern medicine had yet to document.

But then, without meaning to, he shifted.

A sharp twinge shot through his side. His breath caught.

That's new. Is that supposed to happen?

His heart sped up, and his chest felt tight. Has it always felt that way? He tried to take a deep breath, but focusing on it too much made him think he was doing it all wrong. A knot twisted in his stomach. Was that nausea? No, wait, maybe hunger? Or panic? Maybe it was some terrible combination of the three? His fingers tingled. His palms felt sweaty. Oh, great, was this poor circulation? A heart attack? A nervous breakdown?

His brain wasn't interested in reasonable explanations. It was in full disaster mode. *Blood clot. Infection. Internal bleeding. Sepsis. Organ failure.* The words ping-ponged through his skull like an unwelcome game of medical bingo.

He grabbed his phone. Should he call the doctor? Would they roll their eyes at yet another post-op patient convinced they were dying? Or worse, would they insist he come in? Would they scold him for not reaching out *sooner*?

A fresh wave of panic hit him. His stomach flipped, and his vision blurred. As his throat tightened, he wasn't sure if he was breathing too fast or not at all. His body felt wrong, and his mind was unraveling. He was seconds away from either passing out or googling, "How to survive a full-body meltdown."

And then, just like that, everything went quiet.

It wasn't the comforting, peaceful, and meditative kind. No, this was the heavy, all-consuming silence of fear taking up every inch of his brain, squeezing out logic, reason, and the ability to function like a normal human.

In that oppressive silence, a single, awful thought surfaced. *What if this is my life now? What if I never feel okay again?*

This wasn't about pain anymore. It wasn't even about surgery. It was about the fear of never feeling normal again. Of waking up every day with this gnawing, suffocating panic and wondering if he'd ever trust his own body again.

WHAT IS FEAR?

Fear skips the gentle approach and bulldozes through, plants itself in your mind, and refuses to leave. It doesn't care if you're already overwhelmed; it will keep feeding you worst-case scenarios like an overzealous conspiracy theorist. And when you're healing, fear has a field day. Every ache, twinge, and unfamiliar sensation turns into a full-blown interrogation where you ask yourself, *What if this never gets better? What if something's wrong? What if this is just how I am now?*

Fear doesn't wait for proof. It jumps straight to the worst possible outcome and convinces you it's inevitable. Rather than whispering, it shouts and nags, looping the same terrifying thoughts on repeat until you start to believe them. Just when you think you've quieted it down, anxiety chimes in with a new list of concerns you hadn't even considered yet.

Fear is meant to protect us. It's wired into our brains to keep us alive and ensure survival, like when you see a shadow in a dark alley and instinctively decide to walk faster. That's useful. But when you're recovering from surgery or an injury, fear isn't responding to an actual life-or-death situation. It's fixating on all the unknowns and freaking out.

Then there's anxiety: fear's overthinking, and an over-caffeinated cousin. If fear is the "Oh shit!" moment, anxiety is the lingering sense of doom that follows. It's the mind's way of trying to predict the worst-case scenario. Your mind wants you to believe that if you prepare for disaster, you can somehow control it. Except you can't. Anxiety lies, and it's a very convincing liar.

So, here you are. Your body is trying to heal while your mind spirals, and every normal recovery sensation feels like a red flag. Pain shoots through you with every slight movement, and anxiety screams, "You've torn something! Permanent damage! You'll never walk again!" Meanwhile, your body says, "*Calm down*, I'm literally just healing." But logic doesn't matter when fear takes the wheel.

Recovery is full of unknowns, and your brain *hates* unknowns. Every twinge, ache, or weird sensation becomes a guessing game. *Is this normal? Am I dying? Did they forget something inside me?* No one hands you a detailed guidebook that tells you exactly what will happen every single day. The worst part comes when you're waiting, not knowing, and feeling like you have zero control over what comes next.

And speaking of control, let's talk about how healing rips that away from you. Your body, which used to do things without question, now has a mind of its own. You can't move the way you want or find a comfortable position. *Powering through it* like other challenges won't work. Your brain is screaming, "Go! Fix it! Do something!" but your body is like, *"Nah, we need time. Sit down."* And that's absolutely maddening.

Here's the truth, fear is a liar. It's dramatic. It loves to convince you that you're stuck, that this is your forever, and that something is terribly wrong. But fear has no insight into the future. It only knows how to make you panic. Fear is simply noise. It is loud, exhausting, and anxiety-inducing.

Healing is more than physical; it's also mental. Just as your body repairs itself, your mind must learn to work through uncertainty without losing its composure. Instead of fearing pain, remind yourself it's part of the process. Instead of dreading setbacks, accept that healing is messy and *never* linear. Instead of letting your brain spiral into worst-case scenarios, focus on what is actually happening, not the stories that fear is trying to tell you.

Fear can make you feel like you're stuck. But you're not. You're moving forward, moment by moment, whether it *feels* like it or not. Healing is happening. Not only in your body, but in your mind. Fear doesn't get to decide how this ends. You do.

WHY FEAR HAPPENS

Fear is the body's built-in alarm system. Traumatic events like injuries, surgeries, illnesses, or accidents cause your brain to flip the switch into survival mode. It floods you with adrenaline, sharpens your awareness, and prepares you for danger. The problem is, even after the immediate threat is gone, your mind doesn't just return to normal. It lingers in that hyper-aware state, scanning for any sign of danger, convinced that the worst isn't over. This is why, even when your doctor tells you that things are healing well, your brain still whispers, "But what if they missed something?"

Fear doesn't just show up after a traumatic event. It camps out, drinks all your emotional energy, and won't leave. It replays worst-case scenarios, makes you second-guess every twinge of discomfort, and convinces you that something must be wrong if you're not *feeling* better every single day. It's exhausting. And let's not forget about nighttime, when fear and anxiety do their best work.

It's 2 a.m., you're lying in bed wide awake, and your mind is running a full diagnostic scan on your body. Every little ache feels suspicious. Every sensation feels magnified in the quiet. And what do you do? You reach for your phone and start searching for symptoms online, which, as we all know, is always a mistake. One minute you're checking if soreness is normal, and the next minute you're convinced you have some rare, incurable disease. Stop. Step away from the search bar. No good has ever come from a late-night WebMD deep dive.

Fear thrives on uncertainty, and healing is full of it. Healing isn't always straightforward. Some days, you feel better. Other days, you wake up feeling like you've gone backward. Fear loves to convince you that a bad day equals permanent damage and that slow progress means failure. But that's not how healing works.

This stage happens because your brain is trying to make sense of something unpredictable. It wants certainty, but healing refuses to follow a neat, predictable timeline. Every unfamiliar sensation and unexpected fatigue becomes a reason to panic when, in reality, it's part of the process.

And then there's the lack of control. During the worst times of the trauma, whether it was due to injury, surgery, or illness, you were in survival mode with no other choice. Now that the pain is easing, you expect to feel more in control. Yet, your body still moves at its own frustratingly slow pace. You want to push forward, but your body tells you to slow down. And when you don't feel like you're in control, fear swoops in to fill the gaps, making you question everything.

Here's what you need to remember. Just because fear is loud doesn't mean it's right. Just because anxiety is convincing doesn't mean it's telling the truth. This stage isn't a sign that something is wrong. Rather, it means your mind is catching up with what your body has been through. Fear and uncertainty aren't proof of failure; they are proof that you care, that you're aware, and that you're *human*.

Fear wants you to believe that you're stuck and that you'll never feel normal again. But you're not broken. Healing is happening, even when you can't see it. Even when you don't *feel* it. Even when fear is screaming otherwise.

This stage won't last forever. Just like pain, fear will pass. And when it does, you'll see that you were never stuck. You were moving forward all along.

COMMON STRUGGLES IN THIS STAGE

Fear can take over your mind, making you doubt everything. This stage is brutal because it changes how you experience healing. Every normal sensation turns into a potential warning sign, and every moment of tiredness turns into a reason to panic, and every setback turns into what feels like failure. The mind becomes its own worst enemy, throwing obstacles in your path that weren't there before.

Hyperawareness is one of the biggest struggles during this stage. The pain might not be as intense anymore, but now every ache or strange sensation sends your brain into overdrive. You become hyperaware of every sensation that gets magnified as you suddenly notice tightness, tingling, pulling, and stiffness. Instead of trusting that it's part of the healing process, your brain overreacts.

Then there's the dreaded Google spiral. You know exactly what this is. The moment fear takes hold, you grab your phone and start searching. *Is it normal to feel XYZ after surgery? When does this symptom go away? What if I still feel pain after three weeks?* At first, you're just looking for reassurance, but then you click on an article that mentions *rare complications*, and suddenly, you're three pages deep into reading medical horror stories. Unfortunately, the internet is full of worst-case scenarios because people don't go online to post about normal recoveries. They post when they are scared, just like you, which means you end up reading about the most terrifying stories. And yet, fear makes it almost impossible to stop searching, even when you know it's making things worse.

Healing was supposed to feel like progress, but sometimes it feels more like waiting. You wake up expecting to feel better, but instead, you feel stuck. The timeline in your head doesn't match what your body is doing. Some days, you think you're finally turning a corner, only to wake up feeling worse the next day. Maybe you had one good day, moved a little more, and now everything feels stiff and sore again.

This stage also takes an emotional toll. Fear and anxiety do more than mess with your thoughts. They drain you. One moment, you feel optimistic. The next, something small throws you into a spiral of frustration and doubt. The ups and downs are exhausting, and worst of all, they make you feel alone. It's hard to explain this fear to people who haven't experienced it. You don't want to sound dramatic, so you keep it to yourself. But inside, you constantly battle thoughts like, *What if this never ends? What if I don't get back to normal? What if I'm just weak for feeling like this?*

Remember, you're not weak. You're healing.
And healing is hard, not just for your body but for your mind.

The hardest part of this stage is remembering that fear does not equal truth. Just because anxiety is loud doesn't mean it's right. Just because healing is slow doesn't mean it's not happening.

Instead of fighting fear, acknowledge it. It's there because you care. It's there because you have been through something hard. But it's not in charge.

Every time fear tells you something is wrong, ask yourself: *Is this actually happening, or am I just afraid it could happen? Is this thought based on facts, or is it just my brain trying to find control? If a friend told me this, what would I say to reassure them?* Most importantly, remember this. Fear doesn't get to decide how your healing goes. You do. You are still moving forward, even when it doesn't feel like it. You are still healing, even when your mind tries to convince you otherwise. And one day, you will look back and realize that fear was wrong. You were never stuck. You were just in the messy, uncomfortable middle of something that would eventually get better.

RECOVERY STRATEGIES IN THIS STAGE

Fear and anxiety will try to convince you that you are powerless in your healing, but that's not the truth. You are healing, and there are effective ways to take back control. There are ways to quiet the noise, manage uncertainty, and move through this stage without letting fear run the show.

The more you fight fear, the louder it gets. Instead of trying to push it down, acknowledge it. Say it out loud if you need to, "I'm scared right now. I'm worried this feeling will never go away. I'm afraid I'm not healing fast enough." Next, remind yourself that fear is a reaction, not a fact. Just because you feel afraid doesn't mean you're in danger. Fear is your brain trying to make sense of the unknown. Recognizing it takes away some of its power.

Anxiety thrives on worst-case scenarios. It will throw terrifying thoughts at you and make them feel like the absolute truth. What if I never get better? What if this pain means something is wrong? What if I'm not healing properly? When these thoughts pop up, take a step back and question them. Is this fear talking, or is there actual evidence to support this? Instead of spiraling, remind yourself, "I have no proof that something is wrong. My body is healing, and this discomfort is part of the process." When fear loses its grip on your thoughts, you start regaining control.

You already know that googling symptoms in the middle of the night leads to nothing but panic. And yet, it's one of the hardest habits to break. The next time you feel the urge to search, stop and ask yourself, "Am I looking for reassurance or trying to confirm my worst fear?" If you need reassurance, remind yourself that true reassurance comes from trusted medical professionals and personal experience, not from the internet. Step away from the search bar. No one has ever googled their way out of anxiety.

Fear is loudest when you feel powerless. Instead of dwelling on things you don't know or how long healing will take, shift your focus to what you can do right now. You can rest. You can nourish your body. You can move gently, breathe deeply, and remind yourself that healing is happening, even when you can't see it. You're not just waiting to heal; you're actively recovering every single day.

If fear and anxiety keep taking over your day, give them their own time slot. Set aside ten to fifteen minutes each day to acknowledge them. Set a timer on your phone. When it buzzes, say to yourself out loud, "Worry time is over. The rest of today is for healing." If anxious thoughts arise later, jot them down and say to yourself, "I'll think about this tomorrow at worry time." It sounds absurd, but your brain will really begin to work with this boundary. It teaches your brain that fear doesn't get to dominate every moment.

Fear can feel isolating, like no one else could possibly understand what you're going through. But healing is a universal experience, and you're not alone. Find someone you trust, whether it's a friend, family member, or an online support group, and talk about it. Say the scary things out loud. Allow someone to reassure you that your feelings are normal, that they have been there too, and that you will through this.

Affirmations may seem simple, but they help retrain your brain. Fear reinforces negative thoughts until you start to believe them, so counteract this by repeating the truth until you begin to believe it. "Fear is not in control. I'm in control. I'm healing, even when it doesn't feel like it. Just because I feel fear doesn't mean something is wrong. My body knows how to heal, and I trust the process. This is temporary. I won't feel like this forever." The more you remind yourself of these truths, the less power fear has over you.

Fear wants to convince you that you need to have everything figured out right now. It makes you think ten steps ahead, worrying about things that may never happen. But healing doesn't happen in the future; it happens in the now. Take it one day at a time. If a full day feels overwhelming, take it one hour at a time. If an hour is too much, focus on one breath at a time. Right now, you are safe. You are healing. That's all that matters.

This stage is just another part of the process, and just like the pain, it will pass. One day, you'll look back and realize fear had it wrong all along. You were healing the whole time.

FINAL THOUGHTS

Fear can make you feel like you're stuck and can make you believe that healing isn't happening, making you think that something must be wrong. Fear will whisper worst-case scenarios in your ear and convince you that every ache is a sign that something has gone wrong. But fear is just noise, not the truth.

Healing isn't just about feeling better every single day. It's about trusting that even on the hardest days, when progress feels invisible, your body is still working and your mind is still adjusting.

You're still moving forward.

You don't have to be fearless or have everything figured out. You just have to keep going. Recovery includes both setbacks and breakthroughs, and your emotions about both will shift constantly. There will be moments of doubt, frustration, and times when you wonder if you'll ever feel normal again. But those moments will pass.

One day, you'll wake up and realize that fear no longer has a grip on you. You'll notice that you're no longer overthinking every sensation. You'll find yourself doing things you were once afraid to do. And you'll look back at this time and see it for what it was: a season of uncertainty that you survived.

You're not broken. You're healing. Even when healing feels slow or impossible, it's still happening. One breath, one step, one moment at a time.

Fear is not truth. It is the mind's way of trying to protect you from the unknown. It fills the quiet with questions, turns every sensation into doubt, and convinces you that something is wrong. But fear does not know your strength. It cannot see the healing already taking place. You are not stuck. You are becoming. Even in the stillness and not knowing, healing is happening. Fear doesn't get to decide how this ends. You do.

JOURNAL PROMPT: Reframing Fear and Taking Back Control

Fear thrives in uncertainty, making you question everything: your progress, your healing, your ability to move forward. It convinces you that you are powerless, stuck in the unknown. But fear is just a reaction, not a fact. Shifting your mindset can help you take back control.

1. What is my biggest fear right now, and how can I reframe my thinking to regain control?
2. What is fueling my fear? Is it uncertainty, discomfort, frustration, or the fear of the unknown?
3. How can I remind myself that fear doesn't predict the future; it only reflects my worries at this moment?
4. What words or affirmations can I use to shift my perspective when anxiety takes hold?

Instead of "What if I never get better?" try, "Healing is happening, even when I can't see it." Instead of "I feel completely powerless," remind yourself, "I may not control everything, but I can control how I respond." Instead of "This fear will never go away," focus on "Fear is temporary, and I'll move through it."

Write it down. Acknowledge the fear, but do not let it define you. Fear can only keep you captive for so long before it morphs into something more active, more combustible. When worry and anxiety have worn out their welcome, when you're sick of being helpless and scared, that's when the fire begins to kindle. The very energy that once powered your fear now craves action, and when action seems impossible, it turns to rage.

3

<u>Anger</u>

The Battle with Progress & Limitations

The most minor things set her off these days.

The way the sheets twisted around her legs when she tried to shift positions, as if even the fabric was conspiring against her. The dull ache in her back that never seemed to go away, no matter how she adjusted. The sharp, electric sting shot through her ribs if she moved too fast. Or worse, if she didn't move at all.

Even breathing pissed her off.

She clenched her fists at her sides, feeling the warmth of her own palms, the tension creeping up her arms, the heat crawling up her neck. She was furious.

At herself. At her body. At every person who had told her to be patient. Patience? Patience was for people who had a choice.

She had expected pain. She had anticipated discomfort. She had even braced herself for some level of frustration. But this? This constant, simmering, all-consuming rage?

She hadn't seen that coming at all.

It was there in the way her heart pounded every time she tried to do something simple, something that used to be effortless. It was there in the way her throat tightened with every failed attempt at independence. It was there in the way she wanted to throw things just to hear something shatter, to have something outside of her break for once instead of just her.

She reached for the water bottle on the tray beside her bed, moving too quickly. A sharp, searing pain ripped through her side, forcing her to stop. Her hand hovered inches away from the bottle. Defeated. Weak.

Her jaw locked, and her fingers clawed into the sheets as fury boiled in her stomach. She glared at the water bottle like it had personally wronged her.

Maybe it had.

It seemed to mock her, sitting there in all its plastic, half-empty arrogance, daring her to reach for it again. Taunting her.

How had her life come to this?

She had done everything she was supposed to. Followed every instruction, listened to the doctors, and prepared herself mentally and physically. She had planned for the recovery and convinced herself she was strong enough to handle whatever came next.

And still, her body refused to cooperate.

The rage bubbled up before she even realized what she was doing. Her fingers closed around the water bottle, and with a grunt of effort, she hurled it across the room.

It wasn't as satisfying as she had hoped.

The damn thing barely made it past the foot of the bed before it flopped to the floor with a pathetic little thud.

That pissed her off even more.

She slumped back against the pillows, breathing heavily, her pulse pounding in her ears. What a pathetic display of anger. She couldn't even throw something properly.

Tears burned behind her eyes, but she swallowed them down. No. She wouldn't cry. She was infuriated, not sad.

Grabbing her phone from the bedside table, she scrolled mindlessly through social media, her thumb moving faster and more frantically with every new post she saw.

A friend on vacation, sun-kissed and glowing on a beach somewhere. Screw her.

A woman she barely knew was posting about her "post-workout endorphin rush." Must be nice. Some influencer giggling over her morning smoothie. Shut up. Shut up. Shut up.

Her blood boiled. Why was everyone so damn happy?

Did they not realize how unfair this was? How was she stuck here, in this stupid bed, in this stupid body, feeling like a prisoner in her own skin?

She slammed her phone down, screen facing the mattress, as if that would somehow erase the existence of everyone else's joy.

Her jaw clenched when she heard footsteps approaching.

"Do you need anything?" her husband asked, his voice gentle, cautious.

Something inside her snapped.

Do you need anything?

She needed her body to work. She needed to stop feeling so useless, so helpless, so weak. She needed to escape this endless loop of pain, waiting, and more pain.

She did not need to feel like this.

But her husband couldn't give her that. No one could.

She forced herself to inhale, then exhale. Slow, controlled breaths. She clenched the sheets, and her nails dug into her palms. She wanted to snap at him, to scream, to tell him to stop asking stupid questions that had no answers.

Instead, she shook her head.

Because the truth was, this wasn't anyone's fault.

Not his. Not the doctors'. Not the nurses' or the physical therapists' or the surgeons' or the world's.

It was hers.

Her body. Her burden. Her battle.

And that only made her angrier.

She turned her head away, staring at the ceiling, at the spot where the paint cracked just slightly at the corner. She hated that crack.

She hated everything.

Her husband lingered in the doorway for a moment before stepping away, leaving her alone with her thoughts, her useless body, and the water bottle mocking her from the floor.

She thought about asking him to pick it up, but she didn't. Instead, she reached for it. Pain shot through her side as she stretched, her muscles shrieking in protest. She bit down on her lip so hard she tasted blood.

Her fingers brushed the bottle, barely shifting it. For a second, she almost gave up.

Almost.

But anger was a stubborn thing.

With a growl of frustration, she forced herself forward, ignoring the searing ache, refusing to let the pain win. And finally, her fingers wrapped around the plastic.

She exhaled, collapsing back onto the pillow, clutching the stupid bottle like it meant something. And then, just like that, the dam broke.

Tears spilled over, hot and relentless, her body shaking with sobs so deep they made her chest ache. The pain. The fear. The guilt. For days, weeks, maybe longer, guilt had been pressing down on her.

And she let it.

She cried for what she had lost. For how unfair it was. For how much she hated this version of herself. For how, despite doing everything right, she still ended up here. As the tears fell, the anger remained. That was the worst part.

She could cry and grieve, but there was no relief, just exhaustion.

And the unshakable, suffocating weight of having no control.

WHAT IS ANGER?

Healing is often seen as a steady climb from pain to relief, from weakness to strength, from injury to wholeness. In reality, it's unpredictable. One day, you wake up feeling almost normal, thinking, Finally, I'm turning a corner. You move around and do something brave, like putting on jeans instead of sweatpants. The next day, you feel like you've been hit by a truck, your body aching as if no progress had been made. It's infuriating and unfair.

Anger often begins as frustration. This can be directed at your body, at times, or at the well-meaning people who tell you, "You'll get there," while they continue their normal lives. Frustration turns to rage when you realize that determination doesn't speed up healing. The brain may be ready to run, but the body can barely walk, and that's where the war starts.

Anger is more than emotion; it's a survival response, the fight reaction to threats, obstacles, or loss of control. Healing can feel like punishment for something that wasn't your fault, and anger often has deeper feelings like fear, grief, and helplessness. It creates a false sense of control by shifting focus to something tangible. But when anger goes unchecked, it backfires. It raises cortisol, fuels inflammation, slows recovery, and amplifies pain, thereby trapping the body in tension instead of allowing it to heal.

A 2019 study in Brain, Behavior, and Immunity determined that chronic anger increases cortisol and inflammatory markers like IL-6 by up to 40%, directly slowing tissue repair and wound healing (Maydych, 2019). Conversely, a study at the Mayo Clinic found that patients who learned anger management techniques during recovery had 25% shorter recovery times and significantly better pain control, as reported by their own experiences (Mayo Clinic, 2006). The key distinction is that anger itself isn't problematic. It's unprocessed anger that lingers and becomes toxic to recovery.

HOW ANGER TAKES OVER THE BODY

Anger isn't just an emotional reaction; it's a full-body experience. It begins as a spark, a subtle heat in your chest that slowly grows into an uncontrollable blaze. Your heart pounds, a relentless drum inside your ribcage, sending waves of adrenaline through your bloodstream. Your fists clench involuntarily, your jaw tightens, and your muscles coil like springs, as if you are preparing for a fight you can never truly win. The battlefield isn't the outside world. It's your own body, betraying you at every turn.

It doesn't stop there. Your breathing becomes shallow, your shoulders stiffen, and suddenly, you're trapped in your own skin, feeling like a caged animal with nowhere to go. Sleep becomes a fleeting memory as your mind races long after your body begs for rest. You close your eyes, but instead of drifting into the healing embrace of sleep, you replay every frustration, every injustice, every setback. You toss and turn, restless, trapped in a cycle of exhaustion and fury.

And the cruelest part? The very thing that fuels this fire, the overwhelming, uncontrollable need to get better, is the same thing suffocating the healing process. The more you fight, the more your body resists. The more you push, the more it pulls back. The cycle is vicious, and yet, knowing this doesn't make it any easier to stop. Anger doesn't listen to logic. It doesn't care about patience or the healing process. It's raw, untamed, and relentless.

You tell yourself to relax and breathe, but your body resists. Anger is in your head as well as your bones, bloodstream, and cells. It's a storm surging through you, shaking everything in its path and leaving you drained. Still, you're expected to move forward and fight the invisible war of recovery with nothing but sheer willpower and the hope for a better tomorrow.

THE TRUTH BEHIND THE RAGE

People rarely discuss this part of recovery, the way it strips you down to something raw and unrecognizable. The way it makes you grieve for the life you had before.

Anger masks deeper emotions we don't want to admit. The fear underneath stems from the thought that you might not return to your previous state, and that this might become your new normal. Beneath the surface, it's helplessness, the realization that for all the strength and control you once had, your body is now the one in charge. And at the deepest level, it's grief for the independence that's been stolen and for the simple things you used to take for granted.

But we don't know how to sit with those feelings. Society

tells us that anger is intense and sadness is weak, so instead of saying, "I'm scared," we lash out. Instead of saying, "I feel powerless," we snap at the people trying to help. Instead of saying, "I don't know if I can do this anymore," we stew in our own frustration, pushing people away because it's easier to be angry than to be vulnerable.

TURNING ANGER INTO FUEL

Anger during recovery doesn't have to be the enemy. If channeled correctly, it can be one of the most powerful tools for healing. Rather than leading to negative behaviors like self-destructive actions, pushing too hard, giving up, or snapping at loved ones, anger can be redirected positively. It can motivate you to get out of bed on difficult days, encourage you to do that extra stretch, help you practice deep breathing, and help you acknowledge that progress is still happening, even if you can't see or feel it.

This is where anger can serve a purpose. It can push you to take another step when your mind tells you to quit. It can force you to finish that last set of exercises, even when frustration makes you want to stop. Athletes, soldiers, and survivors have all used controlled anger to push through physical and mental barriers, not by lashing out but by channeling it into disciplined persistence.

The body doesn't work on a clock, but it does work for us. Even when it feels like it's failing, it's not. It's healing in ways we can't always see. The sooner we stop fighting against its timeline, the sooner we will find peace in the process.

So yes, healing is frustrating. It's slow and messy, filled with moments of pure, unfiltered rage. But that anger isn't weakness.

It's proof that you're still in the fight. And as long as you're fighting, you're healing.

WHY THIS STAGE HAPPENS

No matter how much you prepare yourself mentally, the reality of recovery often feels painfully slow. The anger stage of healing is raw, frustrating, and deeply personal. Even though you're following doctor's orders, taking your medication, resting, and doing your therapy, it still feels like nothing is changing. And that's infuriating.

This stage happens because progress never feels fast enough. You thought you'd be further along by now. Every day you look for signs of improvement, but the changes are so small they barely register. Friends, family, and even your doctor may tell you that you're doing well, but it doesn't feel that way. It feels like you're running a marathon in slow motion, and every time you think you're nearing the finish line, it moves farther away.

THE "TWO STEPS FORWARD, ONE STEP BACK" STRUGGLE

One of the most infuriating aspects of healing is the inconsistency. One day, you wake up feeling almost normal, you have more energy, less pain, and more mobility. You start to believe you're finally turning a corner. But the next day, it all crashes down. Maybe you pushed yourself too hard. Maybe your body simply wasn't ready. Either way, the pain returns, the exhaustion sets in, and it feels like all your progress was ripped away in an instant.

These setbacks are a normal part of the healing process, but they can be maddening. The unpredictability can feel like your body is betraying you. Good days give you hope, while bad days steal it away. You might start to fear progress itself, knowing that an unexpected setback could follow every small victory. The emotional whiplash of recovery can wear you down, making it harder to stay positive and trust in the process.

COMPARING YOURSELF TO OTHERS

Healing is deeply personal, yet it's almost impossible to resist the urge to compare. Maybe you know someone who had the same surgery or injury and seemed to recover effortlessly. Maybe social media bombards you with success stories of people "bouncing back" quickly, making it seem like you're doing something wrong.

Recovery is not a competition. Everyone heals differently. The factors that affect healing are unique to each person, whether it be age, genetics, overall health, type of injury or procedure, or mental state. But comparison is a thief of joy, and in this stage, it can be one of the biggest sources of frustration.

Social media makes this worse. People don't post the long, painful nights, the tears of frustration, or the moments of doubt. They post the victories. The workouts. The smiling "I'm back to normal" photos. It's easy to forget that behind every "success" post, there was a struggle. You're not seeing the full story, and yet, it's hard not to feel inadequate.

COMMON STRUGGLES IN THIS STAGE

There's nothing quite like the rage of realizing your own body has turned against you. One minute, you're an independent, capable human, maybe even a little invincible. The next minute, you're sidelined, moving at the speed of a sedated sloth, unable to do the simplest things without gritting your teeth in frustration. And the worst part? There's no way out. You're stuck in this body, whether you like it or not.

It's like being grounded for a crime you didn't commit. You didn't ask for this. You didn't sign up for a body that refuses to function properly. But here you are, a prisoner in your own skin, screaming internally while your doctor tells you, in the calmest possible voice, to "be patient" and "trust the healing process." Trust? Oh, sure. Just like you trust your phone's battery percentage when it says 10% but dies immediately.

You know you're *supposed* to rest and take care of yourself, but knowing this doesn't mean it's easy. Healing sounds peaceful in theory, like a slow Sunday morning with coffee and a good book. In reality, it's a full-blown hostage situation where your body is the captor, and it doesn't give a damn about your plans.

The world keeps moving while you're stuck at a standstill. People go to work, run marathons, and post gym selfies. And here you are, celebrating the fact that you managed to roll over in bed without wanting to cry. Your new reality is full of small, humiliating victories, like successfully standing up without getting dizzy or finally reaching the TV remote that was *just* out of arm's reach for an hour.

You used to breeze through your day without a second thought. Now, getting out of a chair requires strategic planning. Showering? A full-fledged military operation. And don't even get started on sneezing, because when your body is healing, a single sneeze can feel like the grand finale of an amateur wrestling match.

Healing demands patience, but patience is a cruel joke when you're the one waiting. Every second feels like an eternity when you just want to be *done*, back to moving freely, driving, lifting things without wincing, and existing without feeling like your body is actively betraying you.

But as we've discussed, your body is dedicated to your healing. Your body is working for you. Every frustrating, agonizingly slow day is your body putting itself back together. Your body is doing what it needs to do, and the sooner you surrender to that process, the less miserable you'll be.

Yes, you're stuck. Yes, it's unfair. And yes, it's going to take longer than you'd like. But one day, you'll wake up and realize that things don't feel quite as rough as they did yesterday. The following day, it might feel a little easier. And eventually, before you even notice, you'll be free from this prison and back to living. *Really* living.

Until then, take the damn nap.

LIMITS AND LASHING OUT

Anger needs somewhere to go, and when you're healing, it lands on whoever is closest. The people who love you the most? Yeah, they're first in line. You don't mean to be a jerk, but when they hit you with another round of "You're doing great!" or "Just give it time!" it takes everything in you not to scream. You know they mean well, but it doesn't make it any less infuriating. Because in your head, you're not doing great. You're struggling. You're exhausted. And you're sick of time moving at the speed of a damn glacier.

Then there are the doctors. The ones you rationally know are helping but emotionally want to strangle. They give you timelines that sound like a cruel joke. They tell you, "This is normal," while you're barely holding it together. You want them to have some magic fix, some better answer. But instead, they tell you to rest and wait. You don't want to wait. You want your body back. You want your life back. And yet, no matter how hard you push, the only response your body gives is a big, fat *NOPE.*

Healing isn't a test of strength. It's a process that doesn't respond to your frustration. Your body is fighting for you, not against you.

So be pissed. Be frustrated. Yell if you need to. Just don't let it turn you into someone you don't recognize. And for the love of all things holy, maybe cut some slack to the poor souls just trying to help you through it.

One of the biggest triggers for anger in healing is the loss of independence. You might miss work, hobbies, exercise, or even basic daily activities you once took for granted. Watching other people live their normal lives while you're stuck in recovery can be infuriating.

It's frustrating to need help with things you used to do effortlessly. Having to rely on others for longer than expected can make you feel like a burden, even when your loved ones are happy to support you. This loss of autonomy can make you feel helpless, and helplessness often gives way to anger.

RECOVERY STRATEGIES: HOW TO CHANNEL ANGER

Healing can be a brutal experience that disrupts our routines and overall well-being. Some days, you wake up feeling almost normal, like maybe you're finally getting your life back. And then, without warning, you're hit with a wave of exhaustion, pain, or frustration that drags you right back down. It's in these moments that anger digs its claws in the deepest.

You have to remind yourself, one bad day does not erase the good ones.

A setback is not a failure. It's part of the process. It's your body screaming, *I'm still working on this.* When you look back weeks or even months from now, you'll see progress not as something measured in single days but as the realization that you're not where you were.

There will be moments that test your patience, that make you feel like nothing is changing. But something is changing. Even when you can't see it, your body is healing in ways that don't always feel obvious. You have to trust that.

LETTING GO OF THE "OLD TIMELINE"

What's the fastest way to make yourself miserable during recovery? Clinging to the old timeline, the one where you thought you'd be back to normal in a few weeks, the one where you imagined yourself bouncing back effortlessly. That version of healing doesn't exist.

Healing often takes longer than you think. The sooner you let go of the idea that you *should* be further along, the lighter you'll feel. Because it's not about "getting back to normal." Normal is a moving target. Normal is different now. The real goal isn't to rewind but to learn to live in *this* moment, even if it's uncomfortable, even if it's not where you want to be.

Adjust your expectations without lowering them. Showing up for yourself, day after day, and doing the best you can with what you have. This can also mean pushing through discomfort, while other days, all you want to do is rest. Both are valid parts of the process.

MANAGING ANGER

Anger is subtle. It doesn't appear as irritation or obvious frustration. Sometimes, it's disguised as irritation with the people around you. Sometimes, it's that overwhelming sense of unfairness that makes you snap at someone who's just trying to help. Other times, it sits heavy in your chest, making everything feel suffocating.

You have every right to be angry. What you're going through is difficult, and no one should tell you how you're supposed to feel about it. But anger that goes unchecked? That can turn into something toxic that slows down your healing instead of helping it.

Start by recognizing where your anger is actually directed. Are you mad at a person, or are you mad at the situation? What it's really about most of the time is the loss, the frustration, the lack of control. But, it's not about them. That's where you need to focus your energy.

Find an outlet. Write it down. Move your body in whatever way you can. Breathe deep, intentional breaths that remind you that you're still here, still fighting. Vent to someone who understands, someone who won't try to fix it but will just *listen.* Give yourself permission to feel it, to sit in it for a while, but don't let it swallow you whole.

What you're doing at the end of the day is healing on multiple levels, physically, mentally, and emotionally. And that means navigating the tough days without letting them define you and reminding yourself that even when it feels like stagnation, you're still moving forward.

You're still here. And that's enough.

FINAL THOUGHTS

Anger is often painted as a negative emotion, something to suppress or overcome. But in the journey of healing, anger is a sign of something powerful, you're still fighting. It means you care and want to heal. You refuse to surrender to pain, fear, or doubt.

Healing can feel like an uphill battle with setbacks that test your resilience. Just because healing is slow doesn't mean it isn't happening. The frustration you feel is proof that you haven't given up. If you're still angry, you're still in the fight.

While patience is often preached as a virtue in recovery, you don't have to be patient all the time. You don't have to sit quietly and accept the struggle, succumbing to defeat. Healing is about movement, sometimes forward, sometimes backward, sometimes staying afloat. And in that movement, even when it feels exhausting, there is progress.

So, let yourself burn with anger. Let it be proof that you're still functioning, still progressing, still rebuilding. Feel the anger. Let it remind you that you are still here, still fighting, still healing. And most importantly, keep going.

Anger shows up when you've had enough. When healing feels unfair, your body won't cooperate, and you're just... done. And it's okay to feel that. It means you care. It means you're still fighting. Let it out. Then take a breath, gather yourself, and as gently as possible... suck it up, buttercup. You've got this.

JOURNAL PROMPT: Reframing Anger and Finding Release

When progress is too slow, when your body does not respond the way you want, when you feel betrayed by circumstances you never chose, anger can drain you, turning its fire inward. But anger is not the enemy. It is energy. Shifting your perspective can transform that fire into fuel for healing.

1. What am I most angry about in my recovery right now, and what does that anger reveal about what matters most to me?
2. Where is my anger directed? Toward my body, my situation, others, or myself. And is that where it truly belongs?
3. How can I release anger in a way that helps me heal rather than keeps me stuck?
4. What words, mantras, or actions can I use to turn my anger into motivation instead of self-destruction?

Instead of "My body has failed me," try, "My body is fighting for me every single day." Instead of "I hate how slow this is," remind yourself, "Every step, no matter how small, is still progress."
Instead of "This anger will consume me," shift to, "This anger shows me I still care deeply, and I can use that care to keep going."

Sorrow has a tendency to turn inwards, to make you wonder not just what happened, but why it happened to you. When sorrow settles in the stillness of recovery, the mind begins its relentless quest for answers, for somebody or something to hold responsible. And often, that leads you back to yourself.

4

Sadness

Grief & Loss of Normalcy

There comes a point in every healing journey where you've cycled through it all, the searing pain, the paralyzing fear, and the burning anger. You've felt every emotion the human heart can hold, and somehow, you're still standing. The pain has dulled, its sharp edges worn smooth by time, but what has replaced it is so much worse.

SADNESS STANDS ALONE

She had been furious at first.

The kind of anger that burned hot and fast, making everything else feel distant. It was as if she stayed mad enough, she wouldn't have to feel the fear, the helplessness, the loss of herself.

She had lashed out at the doctors, at their careful, measured words and sterile optimism. She had snapped at the people who told her she was "so strong," as if it were a badge of honor rather than a punishment. She had been angry at the pity, the reassurance, and the way everyone acted as if healing was a straight line. As if this wasn't the hardest thing she had ever done.

And then, one day, the anger … vanished.

She thought relief would have come by now. But instead of the flickers she hoped for, the small moments where she could forget the weight pressing down on her, even for a second, there was only this emptiness so vast it swallowed everything else.

The pain had dulled, its sharp edges worn smooth by time, but what had replaced it was so much worse.

Sadness and grief.

Not the kind that comes from losing someone else. No, this was deeper, more intimate. This was the grief of losing herself.

The version of her who existed in a world where movement felt effortless, laughter came easily, and she didn't have to think twice about simply existing. She missed the way her body had once felt like home, strong, familiar, trustworthy. Now, every step, every shift, every breath reminded her that something was wrong. Even if no one else could see it, she felt it.

She lay there, unmoving, staring at the ceiling as minutes stretched into hours. Exhaustion clung to her, thick and heavy, but sleep refused to come. Her mind wouldn't let it. What if this were how it would always be?

The thought sent a shiver through her, even in the stillness. What if she never felt like herself again?

She wanted to rewind time. Just a day, an hour. Hell, even a minute. Just long enough to remember what it felt like to roll out of bed without hesitation. To stretch without bracing. To breathe without being afraid of what fresh pain might come next.

The doctors had told her she was healing. That one day, this would all be behind her. The tightness would ease, the stiffness would fade, and the scars (both seen and unseen) would settle into the background of her life. But what if they were wrong?

What if she had been permanently changed?

She squeezed her eyes shut, desperate to escape her dreadful thoughts, but that only made it worse. In the darkness, there was nothing to distract her. No ceiling, no soft hum of life beyond her bedroom walls. Just the hollow, aching awareness of everything she had lost.

She reached down, fingers gliding over the places where her body no longer felt like her own. The once-familiar curves and lines now felt foreign, unsteady, like a puzzle put back together the wrong way.

Tears burned at the edges of her eyes, but she blinked them back. She had cried enough. And yet, even as she fought them, the grief remained, sitting heavy in her chest.

Because this wasn't just about healing, it was also about mourning. Mourning the girl who had existed before all of this. The girl who had never once stopped to appreciate what it felt like to simply be.

And now?

Now, she wasn't sure if she would ever get her back.

WHAT IS SADNESS IN RECOVERY?

Sadness is a shadow. Unlike pain, fear, and anger, this emotion doesn't need to raise its voice or scream like it's throwing a tantrum. Sadness slips in through the cracks, unnoticed at first, seeping into your bones, filling the hollow spaces left behind. It just settles in, quiet and unshakable, until it becomes part of you. It lingers in the silence between conversations, in the weight of an empty chair, and in the way the world moves on as if nothing has changed while you stand there, stuck in the wreckage of what once was. Sadness is patient. It waits. And just when you think you've outrun it, it finds you again, slipping its cold fingers around your heart, whispering reminders of everything you've lost.

Sadness in recovery is different from the sharp edge of pain, the gut-wrenching jolt of fear, the quiet burden of guilt, or the burn of anger. Pain makes itself known. It's the siren blaring through your nervous system, announcing every movement, every breath. Fear is chaotic, an electric current of what-ifs and worst-case scenarios running through your brain at full speed. Anger is more explosive, a surge of heat that floods the body, tightening the jaw and quickening the pulse until even stillness feels impossible. But sadness? Sadness is heavy. It weighs you down, making even the smallest tasks seem monumental.

While sadness doesn't demand action, it demands acknowledgment. It doesn't rush in like a crisis or overwhelm like a wave; it lingers, patient and unyielding. In the stillness, when the noise fades and there's nothing left to distract you, it wraps itself around the quiet spaces of your mind. That's what makes it so damn hard. It forces you to sit with everything that has changed, to feel the burden of what was and what is, and to confront the uncertainty of what comes next.

Recovery, no matter how big or small, comes with loss. You don't have to be missing a limb or relearning how to walk for it to count. Perhaps you're mourning your independence, your ability to move without thinking, or the simple fact that you used to get out of bed without sounding like a glow stick being cracked open. Maybe it's bigger. Maybe it's the loss of a career, a sport you loved, or the body you once recognized in the mirror.

And here's the part nobody tells you: it's okay to grieve that.

People will try to cheer you up. They'll remind you to be grateful, to stay positive and to "look on the bright side." Bless their well-meaning, overly cheerful hearts. But sometimes, there is no bright side, at least not yet. The so-called bright side can seem like a distant galaxy, and you're just trying to make it through one more Netflix episode without crying into your heating pad.

Sadness in recovery goes beyond physical pain. It involves the loss of normalcy, the disruption of your routine, and the sudden realization that simple things like driving, cooking, and putting on socks are suddenly an Olympic-level sport. And no one prepares you for that. No one warns you that taking a shower might require a full pep talk or that you'll miss things you never even appreciated before, like standing for more than five minutes or rolling over in bed without a strategy plan.

GRIEF IS NOT FAILURE

One of the biggest lies we tell ourselves in recovery is that sadness equals weakness. That if you feel grief, you're not strong enough. That if you mourn what you've lost, you're not grateful for what you have. That's absolute bullshit.

Grief is not failure. Grief is proof that what you lost mattered. And feeling the extent of that is part of healing. Ignoring it and pretending it doesn't exist is like shoving a beach ball underwater because it's going to pop up somewhere, probably when you least expect it.

The idea of "grief work" in recovery is backed by decades of research. Dr. Elisabeth Kübler-Ross's model of grief, although initially created for end-stage illness, has been modified for medical recovery by researchers such as Dr. Susan Folkman at UCSF. Research demonstrates that patients who are permitted to grieve their losses (mobility, autonomy, or their "before" body) actually recover more quickly emotionally and sometimes even physically (Stroebe, 2017).

There's no shame in feeling melancholy about what you can't do, what's changed, or how unfair it all feels. You don't have to put on a fake smile and pretend you're not struggling.

You're allowed to sit in the sadness, to acknowledge it, to let yourself feel the full weight of what's happened. Because the only way through it is through it.

THE LOVE THAT CARRIES YOU

The good news? You don't have to carry the sadness alone. There is love in recovery, even in the darkest moments. It's in the friend who texts you even when you don't reply. It's in the nurse who fluffs your pillow when they think you're asleep. It's in the partner who helps you pull your pants up when you can't bend over.

Love appears in the friend who brings you groceries without being asked, selecting soft foods they know will not hurt your stomach. It's in your mom calling every day, not because she doesn't trust you, but because she wants to hear your voice. It's in your dog, who, for some reason, knows to be more gentle, laying their head in your lap rather than leaping up as usual. It's in the nurse who takes an extra minute to explain what they're doing, treating you like a person rather than a patient number.

While sadness is part of this journey, so are love, humor, and the ridiculousness of needing the remote when you're stuck on the couch and realizing you'll have to call for backup. Healing has its messy, frustrating, and sometimes absurd moments. But this experience will remind you of just how much you are loved.

So, let yourself feel it all. The sadness, the frustration, the exhaustion. But also, let yourself notice the love. It's there, even in the heaviness, quietly holding you up when you think you might fall.

WHY THIS STAGE HAPPENS

Everyone eventually experiences the Mourning Period. This is the phase where you realize that healing involves more than stitches dissolving, scars fading, or getting off pain meds. You're also adapting to a new version of yourself. For some people, that realization can suck.

One day, you're an independent, fully functioning adult. The next, you need someone to help you put on your socks. It's humbling, and it can be downright infuriating. It's probably the reason you've thrown at least one remote control or cursed out an innocent cup of water that was *too damn far away*.

You might find yourself staring enviously at people walking effortlessly down the street, like some kind of wistful main character in a tragic movie. Meanwhile, you're stuck negotiating with your body to do basic things, like standing up without feeling like you've just climbed Mount Everest. It's normal, but it can be maddening. Fortunately, it's temporary. Mostly.

If healing had a theme song, this stage would be set to the sound of a sad trombone. Or, maybe the slow, dramatic piano music they play in emotional movie montages. You start off strong, determined, and ready to do everything by the book. You track your progress, celebrate small victories, and convince yourself that, this time, you'll be the poster child for discipline and resilience.

Then, one day, you wake up, look at your physical therapy exercises, and think, *Nah, not today.* Maybe tomorrow. But tomorrow comes, and that "not today" stretches into a week. Suddenly, watching TV for 12 hours straight feels like a tremendous accomplishment. You stare at the water bottle next to you, fully aware that hydration is essential, yet the idea of reaching over and taking a sip feels like an overwhelming task.

It goes beyond sadness into a weird emotional gray area. You're too exhausted to even be frustrated. Sometimes you feel a deep sense of nothingness, like a blank screen where your motivation used to be. You know you *should* care about your recovery, but caring requires energy, and right now, every ounce of that is being used just to exist.

This stage is confusing because healing is both mental and emotional. Your body might be improving, but your mind is still catching up. Even the smallest tasks feel monumental, and no matter how much progress you've made, it's easy to feel like you're stuck in place. You may find yourself withdrawing, skipping check-ins with friends, or brushing off words of encouragement because responding feels like another task on a never-ending to-do list.

It's frustrating, no doubt. But it's also part of the rhythm of recovery. Some days, progress is obvious. Other days, it's invisible. But even if all you do today is exist. That's still enough. As difficult as this stage feels, it will pass.

FEELING LEFT BEHIND WHILE OTHERS CONTINUE LIFE

Ah, the classic "Why is everyone else out living their best lives while I'm stuck here doing nothing?" existential crisis. It's a real gut punch to see your friends going out, coworkers moving forward with projects, or even your neighbor effortlessly walking their dog. Meanwhile, you're over here celebrating being able to take a shower without needing a nap afterward.

Social media doesn't help. Scrolling through pictures of people laughing at brunch while you're stuck on your couch in the same sweatpants for the third day in a row? Unfair. But here's the truth. Life *is* going on without you, but that doesn't mean you've been left behind. You're just on a different timeline right now, one that requires a little more patience and a lot more grace.

When you *do* make your comeback, you'll appreciate those little things so much more. Brunch will taste better. Walks will feel freer. Even work will feel… okay, maybe not that one. But you get the point.

This stage is rough, but it's also important. You're allowed to mourn your old routine. You're allowed to be frustrated. And most importantly, you're allowed to feel *all* of it, just don't unpack and live there. Because this stage isn't the end of your journey, it's just a messy, inconvenient middle part. Healing is happening, even if it doesn't feel like it.

Go ahead and wear the same sweatpants. Have a full-on pity party if you need to. Just don't forget, all this is temporary, and you *will* find yourself again. It will probably be in the middle of a small but glorious victory, like tying your damn shoes without wincing. And that? That will be a day worth celebrating.

COMMON STRUGGLES IN THIS STAGE

So, you've made it past the initial shock, the frustration, and the sadness. Congratulations! Now, welcome to the existential crisis portion of your healing journey. This is where the fun (read:

mental gymnastics) begins.

Ah, the greatest hits of self-sabotage: "I used to be able to do this so easily." "I'll never be the same again." "Was I ever actually that strong, or was that just a fever dream?"

You might catch yourself scrolling through old photos, wondering who that happy, capable person was. Maybe you look in the mirror and barely recognize yourself. And maybe, just maybe, you start spiraling into the thought, *What if I never get back to that version of me?*

But you won't. And that's not a bad thing.

You're not supposed to go back. You're supposed to move forward into a stronger, wiser, more badass version of yourself. Healing isn't about returning to the past. It's about becoming someone who knows what it's like to break and still find a way to rebuild. And trust me, that person is pretty damn incredible.

Just because you can't *see* or feel your progress doesn't mean it's not happening. Your body is working, your mind is adjusting, and whether you realize it or not, you are moving forward. But healing is more like a toddler's attempt at drawing a circle than a straight line. Messy, uneven, and all over the place.

If you're feeling like nothing is changing, take a step back. Look at where you were a week ago. A month ago. Hell, even yesterday. Tiny wins add up, even when they don't feel like much. And quite honestly, progress isn't always measured by leaps. Sometimes, it's just getting out of bed when you really, *really* don't want to.

You start off strong and committed, doing every exercise and following every doctor's order. You push through the discomfort, tell yourself it's worth it, and maybe even start to see small improvements. And then, one day, you just… don't.

You're over it.

It doesn't matter what kind of recovery you're going through. Whether it's from a life-saving surgery, a traumatic injury, or an elective procedure you *chose* to have, the exhaustion still hits. The mental fog still rolls in. Maybe you went into surgery thinking you'd bounce back quickly, only to realize that healing is humbling. Maybe you thought you'd be back at work, back to the gym, and back to *normal* in just a couple of weeks. But, your body had other plans.

What you're feeling isn't just fatigue but something heavier. Some days, you feel drained before you even get out of bed. Other days, you feel nothing at all, like you're moving through the world in slow motion, disconnected from your own progress. The motivation that got you this far? Gone. The determination that pushed you through the early days? Distant. Even caring feels like too much effort, and right now, all your energy is being used just to exist.

And yet, the frustrating reality remains, skipping out on recovery doesn't make it go away. Avoiding physical therapy doesn't magically fix your body. Ignoring follow-ups doesn't speed up your progress. When you ignore these things, your progress stays the same, but your mindset changes. Most of the time, that mindset shift is not in your favor.

You don't have to be motivated every day or be excited about recovery. You don't even have to like it. You just have to show up. Even when you don't want to. Even when it feels pointless.

Even when the end goal seems so far away that you'd rather just nap and call it a day. Healing isn't about perfection but about persistence. Every small step counts, whether you're learning to walk again, regaining strength after an accident, or waiting for the bruising to fade from the facelift you swore you'd never get.

This stage is brutal, mostly because it's long and full of

mind games. But if you take away anything from this chapter, let it be this. You are *healing*, even on the days it doesn't feel like it.

And one day, you'll look back on this and realize that even in your weakest moments, you were still fighting. And that? That's what makes you unstoppable.

RECOVERY STRATEGIES

Sadness has a way of creeping in when you least expect it, making you wonder if you'll ever feel normal again or if progress is just some cruel illusion. It's a natural response to change and loss, but it doesn't have to take control. Moving through this stage requires acknowledging the emotions while continuing forward, even in small ways.

When you're healing, you're also mending your spirit, which can be a struggle for some. It's okay to grieve what was lost. You might be mourning the loss of your independence, former strength, or the ease of doing things without needing a full-on strategy session. That grief is valid.

Keep in mind that you are *not* the sum of what you've lost. Instead of asking, "Will I ever be the same?" try asking, "How can I create a new version of normal?" Because that's what healing is, learning to live in a way that honors where you've been while embracing where you are now.

You don't have to fake a smile or pretend you've got it all together. But you also don't have to hand over the keys to sadness and let it drive. Acknowledge it, feel it, and then remind yourself that healing is about moving forward, not going back, even if it's at a snail's pace.

If you've tied your self-worth to how much you can do, this

part of recovery can feel like an identity crisis. When you can't move the way you used to, work the way you used to, or even *exist* the way you used to, it's easy to feel like you've lost yourself.

Your worth isn't based on how fast you recover, how much you can lift, or how well you can keep up with life's demands. Finding purpose during healing is about shifting the focus from what you *can't* do yet to what you *can* do now. Recovery can be an opportunity to develop patience, find new ways to navigate daily life, and allow yourself the rest necessary for healing.

You are still *you*, just in a different season. And just like winter doesn't last forever (even if it feels like it sometimes), this season of healing will shift too.

WHEN TO SEEK PROFESSIONAL SUPPORT

Feeling sad is normal. Feeling stuck is not.

There's a difference between temporary sadness and something more profound, like depression. It's important to recognize when you might need a little extra support. Healing, regardless of its cause, takes a toll, not only on your body but on your mind. You know the frustration, the exhaustion, the loneliness that creeps in when progress feels slow or nonexistent? Well, it's all real. And sometimes, it doesn't go away just because you tell yourself to "stay positive" or "push through."

If you find yourself constantly withdrawing, struggling to find joy in anything, or feeling like you're in an emotional fog that just won't lift, it might be time to talk to someone. Not just venting to the mirror (though that helps, too) but reaching out to a therapist, a support group, or a trusted friend. Anyone who can help you break the cycle of isolation and remind you that you're not alone in this.

Distraction can be a powerful tool when the weight of recovery feels too heavy. Watching a lighthearted show, listening to music, or losing yourself in a book can pull you out of your head, even if just for a moment. Laughter, even forced, can shift your mood. And if nothing else, just changing your environment can make a difference, even if that means simply moving to a different room, opening a window, and letting the sunlight in.

But if every day feels like you're sinking, if nothing feels enjoyable anymore, or if the exhaustion is beyond what feels normal, it's time to reach out. There is no shame in needing help. Healing is hard, and some days, it will feel impossible. But you don't have to do it alone.

Healing at this stage can feel like trying to watch paint dry. It's slow, frustrating, and almost impossible to notice at the moment. But the trick is to *keep moving*, even if it's just one tiny step at a time.

Acknowledge your grief, but don't let it define you. Find purpose in small victories. And don't be afraid to reach out for help when the sadness feels too heavy to carry alone. Because you *are* moving forward, even when it doesn't feel like it. On the other side of this stage is a version of you who has fought through the hardest moments, learned patience (even if you didn't want to), and come out stronger. And when you do, you'll look back and realize that you never stopped moving forward, even when it felt like you did.

FINAL THOUGHTS

Sadness is about more than loss. It's about change. When we

think of sadness, we often associate it with moments of deep
sorrow, but it's also the feeling that comes with transition,
uncertainty, and the process of healing. Recovery brings
moments of frustration, exhaustion, and doubt. It's okay to feel
sadness as you navigate this journey.

You are still you, even if you feel different right now. It's
easy to look in the mirror and not recognize the person staring
back at you. Maybe you see scars, physical or emotional. Maybe
you feel weaker, slower, or more fragile than before. You may be
questioning your identity now that life has changed. But you
haven't lost yourself. You're evolving and adapting to a different
life.

The goal is not to rewind time and reclaim your old self. That
version of you has not gone through this journey. That version of
you has not fought the battles, endured the struggles, or come out
the other side with new wisdom, resilience, and strength. You are
forging a new path, one that honors your experience,
acknowledges your pain, and carries forward the lessons you
have learned.

Progress doesn't always look like you expect it to. Some
days, moving forward will feel like a sprint. Other days, it will
feel like dragging yourself inch by inch. But every step, no
matter how small, is still progress. Healing doesn't come with a
timeline or a checklist. It comes with patience, with grace, and
with the understanding that you are doing the best you can,
exactly as you are, in this moment.

The hardest part of healing is trusting that better days will
come. It might not feel like it now, but the struggle you are facing
today will not last forever. There will come a time when you look
back and realize just how far you have come. The weight you are
carrying will feel lighter. And when that day comes, you will see

that every tear, every moment of doubt, every ounce of effort was worth it.

If you're feeling depressed, call someone. Call your doctor, your mom, your best friend, a therapist, or a helpline. Heck, even call me. Just don't sit in silence, convincing yourself that you have to do this alone. You don't. You are never alone, no matter how isolating this stage may feel. There are people who care about you, people who want to help, people who will sit with you in the hard moments and remind you that this feeling, no matter how overwhelming, is temporary. This stage will pass. You will get through this. And when you come out on the other side, you'll be stronger for it.

Sadness is a part of healing that no one prepares you for. It hits when things go quiet, when the world moves on, and you're still hurting. It's not dramatic. It just... aches. You don't have to hide it. Missing what you had, feeling the weight of what's changed. That's part of healing, too.

JOURNAL PROMPT: Reframing Sadness and Finding Light

Sadness can feel like a fog that lingers no matter how hard you try to move through it. It settles in when you realize how much has changed, when you miss the things you used to do with ease, or when recovery feels endless. It can make the world feel smaller and dimmer, convincing you that hope has slipped away. But sadness is also a reminder that you cared deeply, you longed for more, and that longing can be the first spark of light to guide you forward.

1. What are three small victories in my recovery so far, even if they feel minor?
2. What moment today gave me even the smallest sense of relief or peace?
3. Who or what helps me remember that I am still supported?
4. How can I honor my sadness without letting it erase the good that is still here?

Write it down. Give sadness space on the page so it does not take up all the space in your heart. Each small victory you notice is proof that even in sorrow, healing is moving quietly beneath the surface.

Sorrow has a tendency to turn inwards, to make you wonder not just what happened, but why it happened to you. When sorrow settles in the stillness of recovery, the mind begins its relentless quest for answers, for somebody or something to hold responsible. And too often, that quest leads you directly back to yourself.

5

Guilt and Doubt

Why Me & Regret

A deep dive into guilt, second-guessing, and learning to accept the healing process

THE WEIGHT OF REGRET

She had managed to sleep in short, restless bursts, waking up each time the pain yanked her back into reality. But this time, it wasn't just pain that greeted her. It was a regret.

Doubt had been creeping in since she woke up, but now it took center stage, wrapping itself around her chest, just as tight as the bandages holding her body together.

She had planned this surgery for years. But now, lying here, trapped in discomfort, her mind replayed every decision that led to this moment.

She recalled sitting in the consultation room, nodding as the surgeon explained the risks. She had told herself it would be worth it.

But what if it wasn't?

Maybe she should have waited. Maybe she should have just

accepted herself the way she was. Maybe she had been selfish, choosing this pain, bringing it upon herself.

Her stomach twisted at the thought. What if she never felt *right* again?

She blinked against the burning in her eyes, swallowing the lump in her throat. She couldn't let herself cry. Not now.

WHAT IS GUILT & DOUBT?

At first, all you care about is survival. The pain, the exhaustion, the endless cycle of meds, ice packs, and restless nights. Recovery feels like a job, one where the only goal is to endure. Then, when you think you're getting through the worst of it, your brain throws a curveball.

Doubt.

Like clockwork, it creeps in. Instead of celebrating how far you've come, your mind fixates on every decision that led you here.

Did I really need this surgery?

Could I have prevented the accident? What if I had done something differently?

It's as if your brain believes that by dissecting the past, you can somehow reclaim control over the present. That if you caused this, you could easily fix it.

But you can't. Yet, that won't stop your mind from trying.

Guilt and doubt often accompany recovery, whether from surgery, illness, trauma, or a personal setback. In moderation, these feelings can encourage reflection and change, but unchecked, they can drag you down. Recognizing and managing these emotions can make all the difference in your healing journey.

Guilt has a way of sneaking in through the cracks of your recovery. It tells you that you should have done something differently, that you're a burden, and that you're taking too long to heal. It makes you feel selfish for needing help, weak for not bouncing back faster, and ungrateful for struggling when others have it worse.

Some forms of guilt are deeply rooted. Survivor's guilt makes you wonder why you recovered when others didn't. Dependency guilt leaves you ashamed for relying on others, even when you have no other choice. Self-blame convinces you that your choices led to your injury, illness, or setback.

While guilt can sometimes be a motivator (prompting accountability and personal growth), more often, it becomes a roadblock. Excessive guilt creates emotional distress, fuels anxiety, and can even manifest physically, slowing down your recovery.

The truth? Healing isn't a test of worthiness. It's a process. And setbacks, struggles, and needing help along the way do not make you weak. They make you human.

Doubt is the voice in your head whispering, *What if this never gets better?* It feeds on uncertainty, past failures, and fear of the unknown.

It can manifest in various ways. Self-doubt makes you question your ability to endure the process, wondering if you'll ever feel normal again. Medical doubt makes you second-guess your doctors, treatments, or procedures, especially if past experiences have left you wary. Future doubt makes you wonder if life will ever return to how it was before, or if you'll always carry the weight of this experience.

While some level of doubt is natural and even healthy, it can also become paralyzing. It can make you hesitate about necessary treatments, resist rehabilitation, and get lost in a cycle of overanalyzing rather than healing.

The key to managing doubt is striking a balance between critical thinking and trust. Educate yourself, ask questions, and seek second opinions if needed. However, it is also essential to recognize that healing requires patience, and not all progress is immediately visible.

Guilt and doubt are often intertwined, feeding off each other in ways that make recovery even more difficult. Guilt can fuel self-doubt, making you question whether you deserve to heal and whether you're doing enough. Doubt, in turn, can lead to guilt, making you feel bad for not believing in yourself or the process.

Overcoming guilt means recognizing when it's misplaced, reframing it with self-compassion, and giving yourself the grace to heal at your own pace. Managing doubt means building confidence in your resilience, learning to trust yourself, and accepting that uncertainty is part of the process.

Think guilt and doubt as markers of growth rather than roadblocks. They are signs that you're actively engaging with recovery. With awareness, patience, and self-kindness, these emotions can become stepping stones, guiding you toward healing and resilience.

WHY THIS STAGE HAPPENS

When you were deep in the worst of the pain, there was no time to overthink. Survival mode took over, forcing you to focus on just getting through each moment. But now that things are slightly better, now that you can take a deep breath without immediate agony, your mind is happy to fill the silence with over-analysis.

One of the biggest culprits of this mental spiral is hindsight bias. Now that you have more clarity, it's easy to look back and think you should have done something differently. Maybe you believe you should have picked a different doctor, pushed for a different treatment, or avoided that one misstep that led you here in the first place. The problem with hindsight bias is that it gives you the illusion of control over something that has already happened. It tricks you into thinking you had all the knowledge and options back then that you have now.

Then there's the comparison trap. You see someone else recovering faster, seemingly thriving, and suddenly, you feel like you're failing. Social media can be a breeding ground for this, with carefully curated stories of people bouncing back effortlessly while you're still struggling to get out of bed. What isn't shown in those posts is the pain, the setbacks, or the quiet frustrations.

Healing is a personal journey, and comparing it to someone else's will only fuel doubt and guilt.

Guilt often sneaks in because healing requires asking for help, and for many, relying on others feels out of character or uncomfortable. Maybe you feel guilty for being dependent, for needing assistance with tasks that once felt effortless. You may worry that you're a burden to those around you, even when they offer support willingly. This kind of guilt stems from a deeply ingrained belief that independence equals strength, when in reality, allowing others to help is also a form of strength. Recovery is not a solo journey and is a shared experience that can deepen connections with those around you.

There's also the guilt of *why* it happened. Maybe you were in an accident and feel guilty for not being more careful. Maybe you ignored a symptom for too long, or perhaps you think you could have done more to prevent this. Your mind craves certainty, so it searches for reasons. It needs anything to make suffering make sense. But not everything can be controlled. Sometimes things just happen, and placing blame on yourself doesn't change the past; it only weighs down your future.

External influences can also make this stage harder. People, even with good intentions, might offer unsolicited advice or opinions that make you second-guess your decisions. "Maybe you should have tried this doctor instead," or "I heard this treatment works better." Their words, even if well-meaning, can add to the doubt you already feel. It's important to remember that your healing journey is *yours*. Others can offer input, but only you and your healthcare team truly understand what's best for you.

This stage of recovery is natural. Your brain is trying to process what has happened, make sense of it, and prepare for what's next. However, it's essential to distinguish between when these thoughts are beneficial and when they may be hindering you. True healing includes both physical recovery and learning how to be kind to yourself throughout the process.

COMMON STRUGGLES IN THIS STAGE

The issue isn't solely guilt. It's also the frustration. Why did this happen to me?

If your injury or illness blindsided you, you might feel like life has pulled the rug out from under you. If it was a sudden accident, a diagnosis you never expected, or a random twist of fate, it's easy to feel like the universe conspired against you. And if it was an elective procedure, there's an extra layer of, *Oh my God, I actually chose this pain.*

Cue the anger, the resentment, and the urge to compare your

struggle to everyone else's. You might convince yourself that you should be recovering faster, growing stronger, or being tougher. Scrolling through social media, you see people who seem to have bounced back overnight. You hear about someone who "barely needed pain meds" or "moving the next day." And suddenly, your recovery feels inadequate. Why am I not there yet?

But here's the truth, healing isn't a competition. Your body, your experience, and your timeline are all uniquely yours. No one else is living in your skin. No one else is feeling what you're feeling. The sooner you stop measuring yourself against others, the freer you'll feel.

Pain leads you to doubt and question, like, "Was this worth it?" or "Could I have just lived with it?" Then there's the ultimate gut punch, "What if I never feel normal again?" The unknown is terrifying, but remember, your body is built to heal. Today may feel like a mess, but in a few weeks, you could feel much better.

You thought you'd be handling this better. Maybe you thought you'd be the exception, the one who breezes through recovery like it's nothing. But here you are, needing help, feeling exhausted, and (God forbid) complaining about it.

And the guilt? It's relentless.

You feel bad for being frustrated, for being in pain, and for not being able to do everything on your own. You tell yourself that others have it worse, that you should be grateful, that you should be stronger.

Let me say this loud and clear: You're allowed to struggle. You're allowed to be miserable. You are allowed to not be okay for a while.

Needing help doesn't make you weak. Struggling doesn't mean you're failing. Pain is not a reflection of your strength but rather a part of healing. Some days will feel like progress, while other days you'll want to crawl back under the covers and pretend the world doesn't exist. All of it is normal. None of it means you're doing something wrong.

Guilt has a sneaky way of morphing into self-blame, whispering thoughts like, "Could I have prevented this?" Maybe. Maybe not. The answer doesn't matter now. You're here and you're healing.

Then there's the classic line, "My body failed me." Nope. Your body is doing a tremendous effort to patch you back up, and instead of cheering it on, you're over here criticizing it. Give it a break. Give yourself a break.

And let's not forget the big one: "I should've been stronger." But hold up, what does that even mean? You are strong. But strength doesn't mean you won't struggle. Strength is getting through all the tough days filled with self-pity and exhaustion. Strength is allowing yourself to feel like crap sometimes while still being there for yourself.

Blame tries to make sense of pain, but sometimes things happen. In those moments, all you can do is move forward.

RECOVERY STRATEGIES

Your body isn't punishing you; it's doing exactly what it's supposed to do, rebuilding, adjusting, and fighting for you. And yet, we sit here beating ourselves up, acting like we deserve to suffer. The only thing you deserve right now is rest, support, and maybe some delicious snacks.

You can't change the past. You made a choice, and now you're healing from it. So instead of rehashing every possible alternative universe where you did things differently, focus on what matters: taking care of yourself. The more you lean into self-compassion, the lighter this journey will feel. It's okay to feel frustrated, exhausted, and even a little dramatic about it all. Just don't let guilt move in and start redecorating your mind with self-doubt.

Permit yourself to heal without shame. If you find yourself spiraling, take a deep breath and remind yourself that this is a temporary situation.

Think back to the moment you made this decision. There was a reason you went through with it. It could be for your health, confidence, or to improve your quality of life. Whatever the reason, it hasn't disappeared just because today sucks. Right now, guilt is fogging up the windshield, but six months from now, you'll be grateful you stuck it out.

So, let's cut to the fundamental question, Do you truly regret your decision, or do you just regret how much this part sucks? Because there's a huge difference. If you're only doubting things because you feel like you got hit by a truck, remind yourself that the car will pass.

Letting go of guilt doesn't always feel like progress, but that doesn't mean it's not happening. Trust the process. Trust yourself. And for the love of all things holy, stop doom-scrolling horror stories on the internet.

Maybe you didn't choose this. Maybe life blindsided you with an accident, an illness, or an injury that flipped your world upside down. And now you're here, trying to piece together a new version of normal while wrestling with the guilt of *What if?* and *Why me?*

First things first, this wasn't your fault. You didn't sign up for this. You didn't ask for the pain, the disruption, or the emotional toll that comes with it. And yet, here you are, dealing with it anyway. That's strength, even if it doesn't feel like it.

Guilt loves to disguise itself as control. If you can convince yourself that this was somehow your fault, it gives the illusion that you had power over it. But you didn't. And that's not weakness, it's just reality. The only thing you have power over now is how you move forward.

Instead of asking, "Why did this happen to me?" try asking, "What do I need to heal from this?" Recovery isn't just about physical healing; it's about allowing yourself to emotionally and mentally process what happened without carrying unnecessary guilt.

Regret is a sneaky little gremlin that loves to whisper *what-ifs* in your ear at the worst possible moments. But here's the thing, regret is only helpful if you turn it into something constructive. Otherwise, it's just dead weight.

Instead of obsessing over the past, ask yourself, *What now? What's the next best step forward?*

Yeah, you would have done a few things differently if you had a crystal ball. That's life. We make choices with the information we have, and then we learn. Regret only has power if you let it sit there and fester. But if you flip it into a lesson instead, suddenly it's fuel.

This experience has taught you something important about your body, your limits, or even how to be kinder to yourself. Maybe it's made you realize how strong you are, even when you feel weak. It might also be an opportunity to show yourself the same grace you'd give to someone you love. Because let's be real, if your best friend were in your shoes, you wouldn't tell them they deserved to suffer. You wouldn't guilt-trip them for struggling. You'd tell them they're doing their best and that healing takes time. So why do you think you don't deserve that same kindness?

Your recovery, no matter how complicated, messy, or frustrating, is part of your story. You get to decide how you carry it forward. Don't let guilt be the thing that holds you back. Let it go. And don't forget to celebrate the small wins, because even getting through a tough day is a win worth acknowledging.

FINAL THOUGHTS

Guilt is heavy, but you were never meant to carry it alone. Set it down. Breathe. Let yourself be free of the weight that isn't yours to bear.

Doubt is normal. It does not mean you made a mistake. It means you're human. It means you care. It means you're navigating the unknown with the best tools you have, and that's all anyone can ask of you.

What healing requires isn't perfection but moving forward, one step at a time. Some days will feel chaotic. Some days will bring frustration, exhaustion, or even tears. And some days, you'll surprise yourself with the strength you didn't know you had. Through it all, you're making strides toward healing.

You don't have to have all the answers. You don't have to rush anything. You just have to keep going. And every single day, you *are* getting better.

And that, my friend, is more than enough.

Guilt echoes with what could have been. Doubt whispers what might never be. But healing lives somewhere in between, in the showing up, in the trying, in the quiet courage of not giving up. You don't have to be certain. You just have to keep going.

JOURNAL PROMPT: Releasing Guilt in Healing

If you could sit down with your past self before your procedure, accident, or illness, what words of wisdom would you share?

1. What would you say to prepare your past self for the hardest days?
2. How would you reassure yourself that healing isn't a straight path but a process worth trusting?
3. What lessons have you gained along the way that you wish you had known from the start?

Use this moment to offer yourself grace, compassion, and encouragement. Your journey is unfolding exactly as it needs to. What would you say to remind yourself of that?

There's a point when you tire of bearing the weight of 'what if' and 'if only.' When guilt and doubt have had their run, when you've played out every last possible means of blaming yourself or altering the past, something changes. Not resignation, a lot more potent than that. The soft acknowledgment that this is your life now, and you do have a choice in how you'll proceed within it.

6

Acceptance

Adapting to the New Normal

THE SHIFT BEGINS

He didn't notice it at first.

The change was so small, so fragile, he almost missed it.

For so long, he had been suffocating under the weight of pain, fear, guilt, doubt, anger, and sadness. It consumed him, defining his existence and closing his eyes to anything beyond it.

The pain was the loudest, stealing his sleep as it gnawed at his bones and wrapped around his lungs like a vice. It dictated every move, reducing him to a man who planned his entire day around the simple act of standing up. He had measured time in the distance between doses of relief, in the seconds it took to move from one position to another without groaning. It whispered to him at night, roared at him in the morning, and convinced him, over and over again, that he would never escape it.

Then came the fear: quieter, but just as cruel. Fear that this was it. That this was who he was now. That he would never be strong again, never be whole again, never be himself again. Fear that this wasn't just a phase, but a permanent state of being. Fear of hoping, because what if he let himself believe he was getting better, only to be knocked back down? What if this is as good as it gets?

And then, there was anger.

White-hot, raging anger that burned in his chest, making his hands curl into fists as he fought the urge to throw something, break something, and scream until his throat was raw. Why me? Why now? He had spent so much time doing everything right, taking care of himself, pushing through, being strong. And still, this happened. The universe had dealt him a cruel hand, and there wasn't a single thing he could do about it. No one to blame, no one to fight. Just his own body. His fate. His war to fight.

And when the anger cooled, the sadness settled in. Deep, aching, and relentless. He wasn't just mourning the pain; he was mourning himself. The version of him that existed before all of this. The man who moved freely, without thinking, without hesitation. He missed that man. He grieved for him. Even though people told him he would get better and that he would find his way back, he wasn't sure he believed them. Because what if he didn't? What if he never truly healed?

The guilt and doubt tangled together, whispering in the back of his mind. Was he trying hard enough? Was he weak? Was he a burden? He had seen the exhaustion in the eyes of those around him, the way they masked their worry, their frustration. He had apologized too many times, saying things like, "I'm sorry you have to help me." "I'm sorry I can't do this alone." "I'm sorry, I'm not who I used to be."

And in the quiet moments, he wondered if maybe, just maybe,

they would all be better off if he weren't here at all.

But today, something was different.

Not better. Not miraculous. Just… different.

When he sat up, it wasn't as hard as it was yesterday. When he shifted, he didn't wince as sharply. And when he pressed his hand to the sore spot that had been his prison, he realized something.

It was still there.

But it wasn't everything anymore.

He let out a breath, a long, slow exhale that rattled in his chest. His hands trembled as he ran them over his thighs, his ribs, his arms. His body hadn't abandoned him. It was trying. Slowly. Painfully. But trying.

And then it hit him.

Like a wave crashing against the shore. Like a dam finally breaking. Like oxygen rushing into lungs that had been too tight for too long.

This is what acceptance felt like.

It wasn't surrender. It wasn't giving up. It was freedom.

For the first time in forever, he wasn't fighting it. He wasn't resisting the truth, wasn't wrestling with what he had lost, wasn't begging for the life he once had. He was in this body, this moment, this step of the journey. And for the first time, he realized he wasn't just surviving it. He was moving forward.

He stood slowly, carefully, but without hesitation. His body still ached, his muscles still protested, but there was something different in the way he moved. It wasn't just a struggle anymore. It was a strength.

He walked to the window and, for the first time in months, opened it all the way.

The sunlight hit his skin, warm and bright, and he closed his eyes.

The breeze brushed against his face, filling his lungs with air that no longer felt heavy. And as he stood there, he felt his future.

Not the past he had been clinging to. Not the version of himself he had mourned. But the version of himself that was waiting ahead.

Whole.

Not because he had gone back to who he used to be, but because he had become something new.

The journey hadn't been pointless. Every painful step had guided him here to this moment, this realization, this clarity.

He let out a real, honest, aching laugh that came from deep in his chest.

He had spent so long fearing this part of the process, this shift between hurting and healing, between grief and growth. But now, standing here in the sun, breathing in the world again, he had an epiphany.

Healing wasn't about getting back what was lost. It was about becoming who he was meant to be.

He wasn't the same man who had fallen into this pain.

He wasn't the man who had been swallowed whole by it.

Although he wasn't himself yet, he was someone new.

Someone who would keep going.

Someone who would stand.

Someone who would walk.

And one day, someone who would run.

And for the first time, that was enough.

WHAT IS ACCEPTANCE?

Acceptance is the moment you stop arguing with reality. It's when you finally realize that no amount of bargaining, denial, or cursing the universe is going to change what is. You're recalibrating and learning how to move forward without dragging around the heavy baggage of "what should have been."

We all have that tiny voice inside our heads that whispers, "I just want to feel normal again." It clings to the past, to the idea of who we were before the surgery, the accident, or the illness. But here's the deal: that version of you isn't coming back. And that's okay. Acceptance is the process of recognizing this truth. Healing means becoming someone new, not returning to your old self, someone who has been through the fire and lived to tell the tale.

Acceptance isn't an event; it's a process. One day, you wake up and realize you're not spending all your energy resisting the reality of your situation. Instead of wasting time wishing things were different, you're learning how to navigate this new version of life. Maybe you've stopped mourning the things you can't do and started appreciating the things you can.

Think about it, when you stop waiting to feel like your "old self," you permit yourself to live in the present. You stop seeing your current situation as a temporary pit stop on the way back to your previous life and start recognizing it as the new normal. What it means isn't that things won't improve, but that you're done fighting the fact that things have changed.

Some days, you'll feel like you've got it all figured out, and then BAM! You'll get hit with a wave of grief for the way things used to be. That's normal. Acceptance isn't a one-and-done deal; it's a dance, and sometimes you'll step on your toes. The trick is to keep moving and to remind yourself that even if you miss the past, it doesn't mean the future isn't worth being a part of.

If you're waiting for the day when everything clicks into place and you feel like you've got it all under control. Sorry, but that's not how this works. Instead, acceptance is waking up every day and choosing to work with what is instead of wishing for what was. It's meeting yourself where you are, scars and all, and deciding that this version of you is worth showing up for.

WHY THIS STAGE HAPPENS

There comes a moment in every healing journey when the war stops. Not because you've conquered your injuries or sickness, not because you've returned to the way things were before, but because you've finally surrendered to reality. And not in a sad, dramatic, violin-music kind of way. It's more like waking up one morning, looking at your body, your pain, your scars, and thinking, "Well, this is what we're working with now."And somehow, that realization doesn't destroy you. In fact, it frees you.

Fighting every single day is exhausting. You start off swinging, determined to claw your way back to the person you were before. You push, you struggle, you swear at your physical therapist under your breath, and you refuse to accept that your body has changed. Whether that change is a newly sculpted body from plastic surgery or the loss of a limb, the battle is the same, trying to fit back into an old mold that no longer exists. But eventually, something clicks. You stop measuring your worth by your former self's standards. You stop fighting the very thing that is trying to heal you.

And that? That's where real recovery begins.

LETTING GO OF EXPECTATIONS

At some point, you realize you cannot force healing. No amount of bargaining, frustration, or sheer stubbornness will make your body bounce back faster.

Your body is not the same as before, but that does not mean it's broken.

Instead of obsessing over what's missing, your mindset shifts to what's possible. Maybe your knee will never let you run marathons again, but you can still hike. Maybe your hand trembles when you write, but you can still tell your stories. Maybe your body looks different after surgery (whether that's a tummy tuck, a mastectomy, or an amputation), but that doesn't change the person living inside it.

Healing is not about returning to what was; it's about adapting to what is.

You may never go back to exactly how things were before. That's the truth no one wants to hear, but hear it you must. Some limitations might be permanent, but they do not define who you are. What defines you is how you move forward despite them.

Humans are among the most adaptable creatures on the planet. We make things work. We adjust, we evolve, we figure out new ways to do old things. That's what healing teaches you: how to work with your body instead of against it.

Maybe your mobility has changed, and walking without a prosthetic isn't an option. Maybe your new body post-surgery looks strange to you in the mirror. Maybe nerve damage means specific movements will never feel the same. You don't have to love every change. You don't have to pretend it's easy. But the moment you stop resenting your body for healing in its imperfect way is the moment you truly start living again.

There's a sneaky little trap in recovery, the comparison game. You remember what you could do before, and every day feels like a cruel joke when you struggle to do what used to be effortless. It's easy to get stuck there, mourning the person you used to be, the strength you used to have.

Just remember that the past cannot be changed. The future, however, is still yours to shape.

Instead of measuring yourself against who you were, you start embracing who you are becoming. You realize that life doesn't end because your body changes, it merely shifts into something new.

Acceptance doesn't mean giving up or showing weakness. It's the exact opposite. It's the moment you stop fighting a battle you were never meant to win. It's the moment you stop surviving and start thriving.

Maybe that means proudly showing off your facelift scars because they symbolize a choice you made for yourself. Maybe it means learning to write with your non-dominant hand because the old one isn't coming back. Maybe it means finally, finally looking in the mirror and accepting that your body (no matter what state it's in) is still yours.

Acceptance is not the end of something old; it's the beginning of something new.

COMMON STRUGGLES IN THIS STAGE

No one warns you that even after the worst of it, the real struggle begins. Sure, the initial pain was brutal, but now comes the part where you have to figure out how to live again, differently.

Recovery does not end when the pain fades. Pain, as awful as it is, is a pretty straightforward problem. It hurts, you deal with it, and eventually, it lessens. What's harder is waking up and realizing that some things may never quite be the same. Maybe you now have a new collection of daily medications that make you feel like an old lady shuffling through her pill organizer.

Perhaps you can't just hop up and go for a run like you used to without your body threatening to quit on you. Maybe you're staring at a fridge full of "heart-healthy" or "low-inflammatory" foods when all you want is a damn cheeseburger.

You don't want to be the person who has to plan around a new diet, set alarms to remember medications, or ask for help when carrying groceries inside. Resisting these changes won't make them go away. You have to learn to work with your body, not against it.

It's incredibly easy to resent what happened to you. It's tempting to play back every moment leading up to your injury or illness and wonder if you could've prevented it. Or worse, wonder why it had to happen to you at all.

Time and opportunities may have been lost. You had to put your entire life on hold while everyone else kept moving forward. That kind of thing can make even the kindest person a little bitter.

And bitterness is tricky because it feels justified. You suffered. You struggled. And now, you're supposed to just let it go?

Yeah, kind of.

Because at some point, you realize bitterness is a heavy thing to carry. It doesn't punish the past; it just holds you hostage to it. You've been through enough. You don't need to make the journey even harder by dragging that weight along with you.

RECOVERY STRATEGIES

There's a moment in every healing journey when you realize no one is coming to save you.

No doctor, no nurse, no well-meaning friend checking in, no

stranger offering empty platitudes. No one is going to wake up in your body, carry your pain, walk this path for you. It's just you. Your body, your scars, your battle.

And that may terrify you. You may wish someone could take this from you, make it easier, faster, lighter. Maybe you're exhausted from the fight, from how unfair it all feels, from how slow and cruel healing can be.

But listen to me. You are still breathing. And that means the world.

Forget what you thought strength was.

It's not about pushing through. Not about suffering in silence. Not about pretending you're fine when you're breaking inside. That's not a strength. That's self-destruction wrapped in pride.

Real strength is softer and quieter than that. Real strength means taking your meds even when you're feeling better, because you've learned to trust the process more than your impatience. It's doing your PT exercises when no one's around, even the tedious ones that don't seem to be doing anything. It's asking for a hand with something heavy rather than proving you can do it on your own. It's the moment you stop trying to rush back to the person you were before and start embracing who you are now. Because, like it or not, you have changed. Pain does that. Survival does that.

Strength is choosing to live in this body, in this reality, in this moment- entirely, without apology.

It's getting up when you don't want to. It's moving, even when it hurts. It's crying, screaming, breaking down, and still waking up the next day to try again. Strength is looking at yourself in the mirror, at the scars, the bruises, the parts of you that feel unrecognizable, and saying, I'm still worthy. I'm still here.

Healing doesn't come in a dramatic breakthrough. No magical moment where everything suddenly feels okay. It comes in fragments, in ordinary moments so small you almost miss them.

The first time you stand without wincing. The day you laugh (really laugh) and realize, for a second, you forgot the pain. The night you fall asleep without fear. The moment you know you're not thinking about what you lost as much as you used to.

These moments? They are everything. They are the proof that, even when it feels like nothing is changing, you are healing.

No one else will see them the way you do. No one will clap for you when you get through the day without breaking down. No one will throw you a parade for showering, for making it to the grocery store, for getting through a meal without feeling like a stranger in your skin.

But you know.

And that's why you have to be the one to celebrate.

Not by making grand gestures. Not by forcing yourself to "move on" before you're ready. Just with recognition. By letting yourself feel proud by allowing yourself to believe that every inch forward matters, even when no one else sees it.

Maybe the most challenging part of healing isn't the physical pain. Perhaps it's the mourning. The slow, agonizing loss of the person you were before this happened.

I won't tell you to stop grieving for them. They mattered. You loved them. You built a life around them. It's okay to miss them. It's okay to feel angry, to feel robbed, to feel like you lost something you can never get back.

But you're still here.

You don't have to rush into that acceptance. You don't have

to force yourself to love the process. You just have to keep choosing to show up in it.

Keep choosing to believe in this version of you.

There's nothing more terrifying than the thought of going backward when you've worked so hard to move forward.

One bad day, and your brain immediately jumps to, Oh no, I'm going back to square one. You feel a twinge of pain and suddenly convince yourself that everything is unraveling. Healing is unpredictable, which can be hard to accept when our brain is desperate for certainty.

Setbacks happen. They are part of the process, not a sign that you're failing. The sooner you accept that, the less power they have over you.

Some days will feel like breakthroughs, while other days will feel like breakdowns. But every single day counts. Every step forward, every stumble, every small victory, all those frustrating moments matter.

What's important is that you continue moving forward. You are still healing, and that's what matters most.

You will wake up some mornings feeling strong, certain, ready. You will wake up other mornings angry, exhausted, filled with doubt. That's okay. That's part of it.

You don't have to love every step of this. You just have to take the next one. And if you need permission to be proud of yourself, here it is.

Be proud that you're still here.

Be proud that you keep trying.

Be proud that you have survived every single day that tried to break you.

You are still here. And as long as you are, there is more life to live.

So breathe. Stand in this moment, in this body, in this reality. And when you're ready, take the next step forward.

That is enough. And so are you.

FINAL THOUGHTS

People often describe acceptance as if it's a finish line, like once you reach it, everything suddenly makes sense. That's a lie.

Acceptance isn't the end of the journey, it's the beginning of a new one.

It doesn't mean you love what happened to you. It doesn't mean you wouldn't undo it if you could. It doesn't mean you wake up every day feeling grateful for the struggle, the scars, the nights you barely made it through. Acceptance isn't giving your stamp of approval for the adversities you've faced. It's finding peace.

It's standing in the wreckage, looking at what's been lost, what's been broken, and deciding you're going to build something new anyway. It's choosing to keep living, not because the past doesn't matter, but because it does, and because you refuse to let it define what comes next.

You don't have to erase the past to move forward. Some pain stays with you. Some chapters never fully close. But moving forward means you stop living inside the wound. It means carrying what you need, honoring what you've been through, and leaving behind what no longer serves you.

The past will always be there. You'll always know what you lost. But you get to decide whether it owns you. You get to determine if you stay frozen in what was or step forward into what can be.

So take the step if it's small. Even if it's slow.
Even Because acceptance is not the end of your story.
It's the start of something new.

Acceptance isn't giving up. It's the quiet moment when you stop fighting what's already changed. It's missing who you were, yet you still choose to care for who you are now. It's not easy. It's not clean. But it's the start of peace, even if it comes with tears.

JOURNAL PROMPT: Reflecting on the Journey

Healing changes you. It reshapes the way you see yourself, your body, and the world around you. Even in the most challenging times, there is something to be learned about resilience, patience, and what truly matters.

Take a moment to sit with your experience. Be honest. Be unfiltered. Write without judgment, without needing perfect words. Let yourself feel the weight of how far you've come.

1. What new perspective or strength have you discovered about yourself and your body through this journey?
2. How has this experience reshaped your patience, resilience, or the way you give yourself grace?
3. What lessons or mindset shifts will you carry forward as you continue to heal?

Let these questions guide you. Write freely. Let your words hold space for both the struggle and the growth. Your story (every painful, beautiful, unfinished part of it) is worth telling.

Acceptance doesn't end with a whisper. It ends with a roar. When you finally stop resisting what is and start working with what you have, something remarkable happens. The energy you spent fighting your new reality becomes available for something entirely new: building a life that's not just different from the one you had prior, but better.

7

Empowerment

Thriving Beyond Healing

OWNING THE JOURNEY – FROM HEALING TO THRIVING

The salt air filled her lungs, crisp and invigorating, as she strolled along the worn path by the coastline. The waves rolled in steadily and strongly, crashing against the shore and tugging at the sand, but never quite taking it away.

She smirked.

God, she understood that feeling.

Acceptance hadn't come easily. There had been months of fighting reality, of raging against what couldn't be changed, of grieving what was lost. But somewhere in that struggle, something had shifted. The resistance had softened. The fight had transformed into a flow.

For so long, it felt like she was just trying to hold on, gripping at whatever bits of herself she could salvage while the rest of her was dragged under. Every time she thought she'd found her balance, another wave would crash down. Another setback. Another impossible moment where she thought, *I can't do this anymore.*

And yet, here she was.

Walking. Breathing. Moving like her body belonged to her again.

She didn't think about her steps anymore. There was a time when every movement had been calculated, a negotiation between pain and progress. She had spent months trapped in her own skin, waiting, healing, hoping. The days stretched endlessly, marked by slow recoveries and frustrating limitations.

She had watched life move forward while she stayed still. And God had that been hard.

It wasn't just the physical pain. It was helplessness. The feeling of being reduced to something fragile, of needing help when she had built a life around being strong. Nights were spent staring at the ceiling, desperately trying to recall what it felt like to be *normal.*

The worst part wasn't the waiting. It was the uncertainty. The terrifying possibility that maybe she would never feel the same again.

And the truth was, she didn't.

She wasn't the same person who had started this journey. And that used to scare her.

Looking at past photos, at the version of herself before everything changed, she could feel nothing but grief. That woman had been fearless. She had taken her body for granted, never thinking twice about the way she moved, how effortlessly she existed. She didn't wake up wondering if she'd have the energy to make it through the day.

For a long time, she had wanted nothing more than to go back. To erase the pain, the struggle, the lessons that came with it.

But now? Now, she wouldn't trade a second of it. Because

without it, she wouldn't be *here.*

Here, she felt her own strength in a way she never had before. Here, she didn't take a single step for granted. Here, where she woke up with a sense of *gratitude* so deep it was almost overwhelming.

She had spent so much time fighting her body, resenting it for betraying her. But now, she touched her scars without anger. She moved without hesitation.

She no longer saw her body as something broken that had to be fixed. It was something that had *endured.*

Chuckling softly, she shook her head as the wind whipped her hair into a tangled mess. A few months ago, she wouldn't have laughed. She would've cursed under her breath, frustrated at something so small.

But now, she found joy in these little things.

The feeling of the ocean air on her face. The strength in her legs as she walked. The way her lungs effortlessly filled with air. The ability to move, to breathe, to exist *without thinking about it.*

That was the real victory.

She had spent so much time focusing on recovery, waiting for the moment she'd finally be "better." But better wasn't a destination. It wasn't a finish line she could cross.

It was *this.*

This feeling of knowing she could handle whatever came next. This is undeniable, unshakable,

holy shit, I actually did this kind of pride.

She no longer feared setbacks. She had lived through the worst and came out stronger. She ate in a way that fueled her, not out of fear, but because she respected what her body had fought through. She moved, not because she had to, but because she *could.*

She was no longer just surviving.

She was *thriving*.

As she turned back toward the path, the ocean roared beside her, wild and relentless, and she felt it deep in her bones.

That's knowing.

That certainty.

That unshakable truth was that whatever came next, she was ready.

Because she had already faced the storm.

And she had *won*.

WHAT IS EMPOWERMENT?

Empowerment (noun): *The process of becoming stronger and more confident, especially in controlling one's life and claiming one's rights.*

Empowerment is so much more than a simple dictionary definition. It's not just about *feeling* strong or *finding yourself* after a hard time. It's not some perfectly polished moment of enlightenment where you suddenly understand the meaning of life and feel at peace with everything that's happened.

No. Real empowerment is raw and messy. It's that gut-punch realization that healing didn't just change your body. It changed you. You realize you didn't just survive the wreckage, you crawled out of it. You survived those nights spent crying, those mornings when getting out of bed felt like running a marathon, those days when your own body felt like a stranger.

You became something more because of it.

For the longest time, healing was the goal. The finish line. The moment when everything would magically return to normal. You spent days, weeks, *months* clawing your way forward, telling yourself that if you could just get through this, you'd be okay again. That you'd feel like *yourself* again.

But then, something shifts.

And you realize: *screw normal.*

Normal was fragile and naive. Normal was the person who took their body for granted, never considering if today would be a good day or a battle. That person is gone.

And in their place?

Someone sharper. Stronger. Someone who doesn't just exist but owns their existence.

Empowerment is the moment you stop trying to go back to who you were and start embracing who you've become.

It's the moment you stop thinking of yourself as someone who recovered and start seeing yourself as someone who rose up from the ashes.

It's waking up, stretching, and instead of bracing for pain, realizing… You feel good. And not just physically. You feel whole.

It's standing in front of the mirror, running your fingers over the scars that once made you flinch, and thinking, *Damn. I earned this body. This body carried me through hell and back. And I love it for that.*

It's finally understanding that healing wasn't about getting back to the life you had before. It was about building something better.

Despite facing anguish, questioning, disappointment, and heartbreak, you've survived it all. And now?

Now, you're done playing small. Done waiting. Done questioning whether you're strong enough, ready enough, *worthy* enough.

You already survived the worst.

Now, it's time to thrive.

COMMON STRUGGLES IN THIS STAGE

Empowerment sounds great on paper. It's strong, inspiring, a moment of triumph. But getting to this stage isn't only a straight road paved with newfound confidence.

There are struggles here, too.

You don't just step into empowerment with a perfectly clear mind and a fearless heart. You step into it, being fully *aware* of your body, your limits, and the reality that life doesn't always play fair.

This stage is liberating, but it also comes with fears, doubts, and a strange kind of *emptiness*

when the battle you've been fighting for so long is finally over.

No one tells you that healing doesn't just change your body, it changes the way you *see* your body.

Before, you moved through life without thinking twice about every little ache or pain. But now? Every twinge, every weird sensation, every unexpected fatigue makes you pause. Makes you wonder, *is this normal? Is something wrong? Am I about to go through all of that again?*

You'll find yourself doing things like poking at old surgical sites, seeing if they still feel "normal." You'll Google symptoms you would have previously ignored, searching your body like a detective for signs that something's amiss. A headache that once meant "I need water" makes you worry it's related to your medication. A good day followed by a tired day has you spiraling into "Am I relapsing?" When friends gripe about minor pains, part of you wishes they could be shaken and told, "You have no idea how good you have it."

You don't mean to be paranoid. You don't *want* to live in fear. But after everything you've been through, it's hard to trust that your body won't betray you again.

And that's exhausting.

It's a weird kind of mental tug-of-war. On one hand, you're stronger than ever. You've been through hell and back, and you know how resilient you are.

On the other hand, you're more aware now than ever. You know exactly how bad things can get because you've experienced it firsthand. This deep insight makes it difficult just to brush things off as easily as you once did.

This fear is normal. It's frustrating, but it's *normal*. The key is realizing that while you may not always trust your body yet, you can trust *yourself*.

You know how to listen to it now. You know when to push, when to rest, and when to seek help. You've already survived the worst. And no matter what happens next, you know you can handle it.

No one comes out of a healing journey the same person they were before. And that's not necessarily a bad thing.

But it's *a thing*.

Maybe your body looks different. Maybe it feels different. Maybe your energy isn't what it used to be, or your priorities have shifted, or the things that used to matter *so much* now feel small and insignificant.

There's this weird expectation that healing means returning to who you were before. That one day, you'll wake up and *finally* feel like yourself again.

That version of you might be gone.

While that might sound tragic at first, it's actually incredibly powerful.

Because the person you are now? The person who survived this, who fought through the worst of it, who learned how to advocate for themselves, who found strength in places they never thought possible? That person deserves to be seen. That person is worth honoring.

It's okay to mourn what was. To acknowledge that things have changed. But don't get stuck chasing an old version of yourself when the new version of you is so much stronger, wiser, and more intentional.

You didn't just heal. You *evolved.*

For so long, healing was the goal. You had a purpose each day, to get through it, get better, and keep going. But what happens when that purpose is gone? When do you no longer need to fight anymore?

There's a strange *emptiness* in that.

Not because you're not grateful to be here, but because healing was your full-time job for so long. And now?

Now, you
have to figure out
what comes next.
And that can
feel… weird.

It's like finishing a book you've been deeply invested in. You turn the last page and sit there, staring at the cover, thinking, *Well… now what?*

This part of the journey is about shifting your focus. Moving from trying to get through this to, "What do I want next?"

Moving forward becomes your decision when you have

everything you've learned to work with, the strength, the resilience, the hard-earned perspective that can create a life better than before.

Not just surviving.

Not just healing.

Thriving.

RECOVERY STRATEGIES

True empowerment means using your struggles as experiences that fuel and strengthen you, rather than simply overcoming them.

Healing transforms into a greater purpose when you shift your focus from what happened to how you choose to use it.

USING THE EXPERIENCE FOR GROWTH – BECOMING AN ADVOCATE OR SUPPORTING OTHERS

You don't go through something like this and come out unchanged. No amount of textbooks, research, or outside advice can replace what your experience has given you through the setbacks, the victories, and the lessons learned in the most challenging moments, lived experience.

Someone out there, right now, is going through the same thing you did. And they feel alone. Just like you did.

They're wondering if they'll ever feel normal again, if the pain will ever stop, if anyone actually understands what they're going through. And you? You do.

You don't have to be "fully healed" to be someone's lifeline. You don't have to have everything figured out to offer someone hope. Sometimes, simply saying, "I've been there, and I made it through," is enough to change someone's world.

Advocacy doesn't have to mean standing on a stage or writing a book (though, hey, why not?). It can be as simple as talking to a friend who's struggling. Joining a support group and offering your story. Sharing your journey online in a way that reminds others that they are not alone.

Your pain doesn't have to be pointless. It can become a lifeline to help someone persevere when they're ready to give up.

MAINTAINING LONG-TERM HEALTH & RESILIENCE

Here's the thing about recovery: it doesn't end.

The worst of it may be behind you, and the pain might be gone, but long-term health is an ongoing commitment.

You know what it's like to lose control of your body. To feel like you're at its mercy, waiting for it to cooperate. And now that you've fought to reclaim it, you don't just *go back* to taking it for granted.

You listen.

You stay mindful of what your body needs, now and in the future. You don't ignore warning signs. You don't push yourself to the point of exhaustion and expect it to bounce back magically. You respect your body in a way you never did before.

This also applies to mental strength. Healing your body and mindset is equally important. Learning to be patient with yourself and letting go of expectations is a crucial part of navigating life's obstacles. Continue to show yourself compassion, even when you are frustrated beyond belief.

That part doesn't stop just because you feel better.

Habits like the patience you developed, the self-care you practiced, and the boundaries you learned to set are part of your resilience now.

And if you want to keep thriving, you don't abandon them. You honor them.

GRATITUDE PRACTICE

You don't have to be grateful for what happened.

You don't have to romanticize the pain. You don't have to look back and say, "I'm so glad I went through that." Because honestly? It sucked. It tested you in ways that no one should ever have to be tested.

But you can be grateful for the lessons you've learned. For who you've become. For the strength you never knew you had.

You can be thankful for the relationships that deepened because of this journey, the patience and resilience you gained, and for the way you see life differently now.

You've learned to appreciate the little things, no longer taking your body for granted, and are living with a more profound sense of purpose.

Gratitude doesn't mean pretending the pain was a gift. Instead, you're acknowledging that even during the challenging moments, growth prevailed.

When you can look back and say, "That was brutal, but I made it through, and I'm better because of *it,*" this isn't just healing.

That's power.

FINAL THOUGHTS

Take a deep breath.

Not because you have to, not because you're checking for pain or discomfort, just because you *can*.

Let that sink in for a moment. You made it.

Not only through the pain, the setbacks, the doubt, and the moments when you thought you'd never feel normal again.

You made it through all of it.

And now you're standing on the other side, stronger, wiser, and more alive than ever before.

Your body may carry reminders of what you've been through: a scar, a memory, a new awareness of how precious your health truly is. But those are not signs of what was lost. They are proof of what you survived.

At some point along the way, without even realizing it, you stopped waiting for things to go back to "normal." You stopped measuring your days in pain levels and doctor's visits. You stopped feeling like a victim of what happened and started *owning* your story.

That's not just healing. That's becoming.

This journey has changed you in ways you never could have expected. You've learned how to listen to yourself, how to trust your instincts, how to take care of your body, not because you have to, but because you *want to*. You've learned patience, grace, and the incredible strength that comes from simply showing up for yourself.

So now, as you stand here, whole in a way you never thought possible, there's only one question left. What now?

And the answer?

Anything.

This life, your life, is yours again.

And you, my friend, are ready for whatever comes next.

Not just healed.

Empowered.

You moved through pain that nearly broke you. Through fear, doubt, and days you didn't think you'd survive. But you did. And somewhere along the way, you became someone new. This isn't just healing. This is becoming. You don't need to chase who you were. You can breathe here.

JOURNAL PROMPT: Using Your Healing Journey to Inspire

Your healing journey has shaped you, strengthened you, and given you a new perspective. Take a moment to reflect on how you can use that experience to inspire yourself or others.

1. What is one way I can use my healing journey to inspire myself or others?
2. How has this experience changed your perspective on life, health, or resilience?
3. Is there a way to help others who are going through something similar?
4. What would you say to someone who is just beginning this journey?

Take your time. Be honest. Let yourself recognize just how far you've come and how powerful your story truly is.

CONCLUSION

There will be moments when it feels impossible, when progress is so slow that you wonder if you're moving forward. There will be days when frustration, sadness, and doubt feel stronger than your belief in your recovery. But healing is happening whether you can see it or not.

Pain doesn't last forever. Fear doesn't get the final say. Frustration will not always weigh you down. You're moving forward, and one day (sooner than you think), you will look back and realize you made it through.

Beyond healing from an injury, illness, or surgery, this journey teaches you how to keep moving forward, even when things do not go as planned. It's about resilience, patience, and the kind of strength that only comes from overcoming something difficult.

So know that you're exactly where you need to be right now, whether it's still being in pain, trapped in fear, struggling with frustration, or beginning to accept your new normal. Healing takes time, one step at a time, until you're no longer just surviving. *You are thriving.*

There are people, tools, and resources that can help. Here are a few ways to stay supported on your journey:

FINDING SUPPORT – YOU DO NOT HAVE TO DO THIS ALONE
- Support Groups: Whether in-person or online, connecting with others who have been through

similar experiences can be incredibly reassuring.
- Therapy & Counseling: If emotional struggles feel overwhelming, talking to a professional can help you work through fear, frustration, and grief.
- Family and Friends: Letting people in and allowing them to support you does not make you weak; it makes you human.

MEDICAL & PROFESSIONAL GUIDANCE
- Doctors & Specialists: Keep up with follow-ups and reach out if something happens.
- Physical Therapy & Rehabilitation: Continued movement and care can help strengthen your body and prevent setbacks.
- Pain Management & Holistic Care: Acupuncture, massage, mindfulness, and guided breathing can all support long-term healing.

NEXT STEPS IN LONG-TERM SELF-CARE
- Continue Listening to Your Body: Healing does not stop when the pain fades. Staying in tune with what your body needs is key.
- Stay Active in a Way That Works for You: Movement looks different for everyone. Find something that feels good and supports your body's needs.
- Practice Gratitude & Reflection: Looking back on how far you have come can remind you of your strength and resilience.
- Know That Growth Never Ends: Recovery isn't just about returning to how things were before; it's about growing into something even stronger.

You are Stronger Than You Think

Getting better doesn't proceed logically. It's usually confusing, heartbreaking, endless, and punctuated by constant setbacks. But every hard day, every moment of doubt, and every small victory have brought you to this point on the other side of something complex.

No matter how long it takes or how many ups and downs you have faced, you're still standing. And that's proof of your strength.

You are healing. You are adapting. You are moving forward. And most of all, you are not alone.

Healing will guide you through pain, fear, guilt, anger, sadness, and ultimately to acceptance and empowerment. Not in a straight line. Not just once. These stages shift and circle back when you least expect them. Let them. Feel them. Grow through them. And if everything feels too heavy, take a bath. Let the water hold what you can't.

RESOURCES AND REFERENCES

Gauntlett-Gilbert, J., & Brook, P. (2018). Living well with chronic pain: the role of pain-management programmes. BJA Education, 18(1), 3–7. https://doi.org/10.1016/j.bjae.2017.09.001

LeDoux, J. E. (2014). Coming to terms with fear. Proceedings of the National Academy of Sciences, 111(8), 2871–2878. https://doi.org/10.1073/pnas.1400335111

Lumley, M. A., Cohen, J. L., Borszcz, G. S., Cano, A., Radcliffe, A. M., Porter, L. S., Schubiner, H., & Keefe, F. J. (2011). Pain and emotion: A biopsychosocial review of recent research. Journal of Clinical Psychology, 67(9), 942–968. https://doi.org/10.1002/jclp.20816

Martin, M. (2024, September 5). Brain scans reveal that mindfulness meditation for pain is not a placebo. UC San Diego Today. https://today.ucsd.edu/story/brain-scans-reveal-that-mindfulness-meditation-for-pain-is-not-a-pla cebo

Maydych, V. (2019). The interplay between stress, inflammation, and emotional attention: Relevance for depression. Frontiers in Neuroscience, 13, 384. https://doi.org/10.3389/fnins.2019.00384

Mayo Clinic. (2006). Comprehensive Pain Rehabilitation Center: Program guide. Mayo Clinic.

Robb-Dover, K. (2023, July 2). Pain & the mind: Anxiety. FHE Health. https://fherehab.com/learning/pain-anxiety

Stroebe, M., Schut, H., & Boerner, K. (2017). Cautioning health-care professionals: Bereaved persons are misguided through the stages of grief. OMEGA - Journal of Death and Dying, 74(4), 455–473. https://doi.org/10.1177/0030222817691870

UCLA Department of Psychology. (n.d.). Naomi Eisenberger. UCLA Department of Psychology. https://www.psych.ucla.edu/faculty-page/neisenbe/

ABOUT THE AUTHOR

For more than a decade, Kenna Kaylee has dedicated her life to caring for patients, loved ones, and anyone navigating the delicate path of healing. Her journey has taken her from operating rooms and hospital rooms to quiet moments at home, always standing beside those in pain, fear, or recovery.

As a Registered Nurse with over 14 years of experience, Kenna has guided countless individuals through surgery, illness, trauma, and the delicate stages of recovery. She has held leadership roles, supported medical teams, and most importantly, served as an unwavering advocate for those who could not find their voice.

Kenna believes that every scar tells a story and that true healing goes far beyond the body. It reaches the heart, mind, and spirit. She has been a steady hand for those who needed strength when their own felt lost, and a compassionate witness to the courage it takes to keep moving forward.

Her passion for healing and fierce dedication to advocacy inspired her to create Kare Health Solutions, where she continues to walk with others through some of life's most challenging moments. Beyond her professional work, she is also a mother and entrepreneur who reminds us that healing is not only possible but also deeply personal, and no one should ever have to go through it alone.